Keto Meal Prep

This Book Includes:

The Ultimate Healthy Collection on Vegan Keto Diet and Keto Chaffle Recipes, with Low Carb to Maximize Weight Loss and Delicious Ideas to Prepare Desserts

By Tyler Allen

Vegan Keto Diet

The Ultimate Ketogenic Diet and Cookbook, With Low-Carb and Vegan Keto Bread Recipes to Maximize Weight Loss and Special Ideas to Build Your Keto Vegan Meal Plan

By Tyler Allen

4

Summary

Chapter 1: What Is Ketogenic Diet and How Does it Work? **11**

How Does Keto Work? 12

What Keto Is and Isn't.. 13

Ketosis and Ketones 15

What Is the Science Behind Ketosis and Producing Ketones? 16

Chapter 2: What Is a Vegan Diet?............................ **17**

Why Is Vegan Diet Healthy? 18

Chapter 3: The Vegan Keto Diet: Why Is it the Most Beneficial Way to Eat? **21**

Vegan Ketosis: How Does Ketosis Work While on a Vegan Diet?..22

Vegan Ketosis: How Is it Different From Regular Ketosis?.....23

The Advantages and Disadvantages of the Vegan Keto Diet ... 24

Chapter 4: Getting Started on the Vegan Keto Diet: Is it Right for You? **27**

Before You Begin the Vegan Keto Diet: Steps to Take............ 27

The First Week of Your Vegan Keto Diet 29

Adapting to a Plant-Based Diet *30*

Going Vegan: Reducing Carbohydrates *31*

Chapter 5: What Foods Can You Eat on the Vegan Keto Diet? 35

Choosing Low-Carb, Plant-Based Foods to Meet Your Diet goals.. 35

Soy *35*

Seeds and Nuts *36*

Chia Seeds... *37*

Mushrooms.. *37*

Dark, Green Leafy Vegetables *38*

Cruciferous Vegetables: Cauliflower and Broccoli............. *38*

Zucchini *38*

Fruits: Avocados, Berries, and on Occasion, Citrus Fruits *39*

Avocado *39*

MCT and Coconut Oil... *39*

Low-Carb Sweeteners *40*

Fermented Food Options *40*

Seaweed and Sea Vegetables...................................... *40*

How to Choose Foods and Balance Your Nutritional Needs....41

Vegan Keto Bread: How to Make it and Add Into Your Regular Meals 41

Vegan Keto Bread Recipe 44

Flour-Free Almond Bread 44

Vegan Keto Seed Bread 46

Simple Vegan Keto Bread..47

Adding Vegan Keto Bread to Your Regular Meals 49

Tools and Equipment for a Vegan Keto Diet 49

Special & Unique Ingredients to Consider for the Diet 51

Chapter 6: Frequently Asked Questions and Answers About the Vegan Keto Diet **53**

How Does the Vegan Keto Diet Maximize Weight Loss? 53

Will I Meet All of My Daily Nutritional Requirements? 54

Is it an Easy Diet to Follow? 54

What Happens if I "Cheat" by Eating Animal-Based or High-Carb Food?.. 55

Chapter 7: Meal Planning and Preparation **57**

First Week: Keeping it Simple..58

Second Week: Adding More Options 58

Third Week: Getting Creative..59

Fourth Week: Staying on Track...59

Vegan Keto Recipes 60

Breakfast...60

Snacks *93*

Lunches *107*

Dinners *138*

Desserts.. *161*

Fat Bombs: A New Way to Treat Yourself on the Vegan Keto Diet... *163*

Drinks *181*

Chapter 8: Bonus Chapter: Enjoying the Vegan Keto Diet and Recipes Without Expensive Ingredients 189

Chapter 9: Vegan Keto Diet for Long-Term Success in Health and Weight Loss Goals.................................... 191

Conclusion 193

Chapter 1: What Is Ketogenic Diet and How Does it Work?

The ketogenic diet is one of the most popular diets today, with many celebrity endorsements, social media attention, and ongoing scientific research to support the benefits of eating keto. Traditionally, diets center around low calories and reducing fat, whereas the keto way of eating works by increasing the amount of healthy fats and reducing carbohydrates. This has the effect of switching the body's main source of fuel from glucose and carbohydrates to stored fat, which produces significant results in a short period of time. Initially, the ketogenic diet appears to be another fad, though historically, it was developed nearly one hundred years ago for the treatment of certain medical conditions, including epilepsy (specifically reducing seizures), regulating insulin, and other health benefits. There were positive results for both children and adults alike—significant reduction or elimination of epileptic seizures and improved cognitive abilities. Weight loss was another benefit of the diet because of the low-carbohydrate intake, which is one of the major reasons that the ketogenic diet grew in popularity. As medications were developed, this way of eating became less common until just recently, with a new surge of health and diet consciousness.

Most people's diets consist of a high level of carbohydrates: bread, pasta, grains, pastries, and sugary foods. These food items are offered at every restaurant, drive-through, and coffee shop, so they are generally difficult to avoid. The ketogenic way of eating aims to reduce the level of carbohydrates in our diets for 100+ grams per day to a mere 20 grams at the maximum. Healthy fats (monounsaturated and polyunsaturated fats) from natural oils and foods are the largest part of the keto diet at 70-75%, followed by protein at 20%, and carbohydrates, making up the remaining 0-5%:

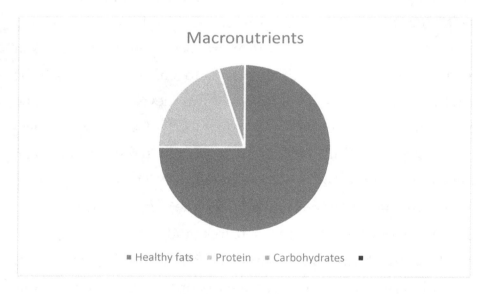

How Does Keto Work?

When your body burns fuel, the first source is always carbohydrates and glucose. With a typical high-carb diet, these are readily available and provide a lot of energy. If the amount of carbohydrates in your diet is high, your body will continue to access this source as fuel, moving to fat stores as the next option, only once the carbs are completely depleted. When carbs are significantly reduced in your meal plan, your body will shift to fat stores. At this point, carbohydrates and glucose are low and used up quickly.

What Keto Is and Isn't

Keto isn't a new concept, nor it is a temporary trend; it is a sustainable, long-term solution for the prevention and treatment of many health conditions, as well as weight loss goals. As with every diet, there have been divisive opinions and reactions to the low-carb way of eating, from adverse health effects to gaining back all of the weight that was lost if carbs are added back into the diet. There are a lot of misconceptions about the keto diet, which can easily be cleared up with a bit of research and reading about the history and studies conducted on this diet:

What keto is

A sustainable, long-term diet for weight loss and maintenance, prevention, and treatment of certain medical conditions

Supported by scientific research and studies from nearly 100 years ago

A nutritious, balanced diet consisting of natural and healthy fats and moderate amounts of protein, with nutrients, fiber, and a small amount of carbohydrates

Flexible, easy to follow, and can fit within your budget

What keto is not

It's trendy and popular, though not just a "fad" diet

Unhealthy. Although the keto diet is not for everyone and may have restrictions depending on your individual medical condition(s), it is relatively safe for most people

Overly restrictive. The low-carb diet may appear challenging, though there are delicious options to replace high-carb foods with healthy, nutritious meals

It's an expensive diet. It can be a challenge to find the right foods, though, with some effort and budgeting, it can cost the same as any diet.

Ketosis and Ketones

Ketosis is the process by which your body becomes adapted to fat, switching to fat as the fuel-burning source. This occurs when ketones are produced by the liver, as a response to low-carb consumption. During the state, you may experience some changes in your body, such as high energy and better mental focus. During your first experience of ketosis, you may experience "keto flu" symptoms, which include fatigue, light nausea, and other flu-like symptoms, though these are temporary and will disappear within the first two weeks. The long-term benefits of the ketogenic diet outweigh the initial side effects, especially adapting to a vegan ketogenic diet, which combines the health benefits of both ways of eating into a sustainable, healthy diet.

Once your body becomes accustomed to ketosis, you'll begin to notice weight loss, high levels of energy, and other benefits. Blood sugar levels will drop as insulin becomes regulated better. Cravings for sugary and processed foods will drop drastically. If weight loss is a goal, you will notice a significant change within weeks or one to two months.

What Is the Science Behind Ketosis and Producing Ketones?

Ketones are produced by the body in response to low glucose levels. This occurs when all carbohydrates and glucose is used up for fuel. The level of insulin will fall, and a process of beta-oxidation begins. Beta-oxidation occurs when fatty acids move from fat cells and into the body's bloodstream, which results in the production of ketones. There are three different types of ketones that become present in the blood once ketosis is reached and maintained. The first ketone created is acetoacetate (AcAc), in the initial state of ketosis, followed by the production of two more types: BHB (B-hydroxybutyrate) and acetone. Acetone is produced less than BHB, as more of a by-product of AcAc, and discarded by the body. When a state of ketosis is maintained, your body will be fat-adapted and continue to burn fat stores instead of glucose. In order to remain in this state and continue to benefit from rapid weight loss, a low carbohydrate level of under 20 grams per day is required. In order to achieve a nutritious state of ketosis, it is important to track macronutrients and make healthy food choices. This book will provide food options, meal plans, and recipes as tools for your new way of eating.

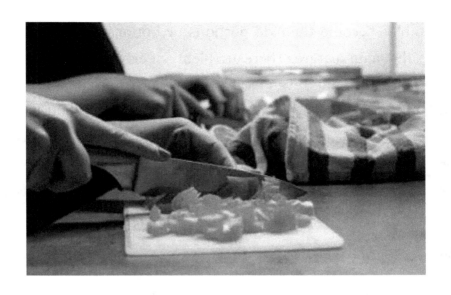

Chapter 2: What Is a Vegan Diet?

The vegan diet is a plant-based diet without any meat products or by-products like dairy, eggs, or any foods that contain ingredients derived from animals. Veganism or plant-based eating is, and continues to remain, a popular and sustainable way of eating for people all over the world, for a variety of reasons: religious, environmental, ethical, or for better health. It is a beneficial way of eating, as it reduces many conditions caused by animal products, such as high cholesterol, heart disease, cardiovascular problems, and weight gain.

A plant-based diet contains much more variety and taste than many people think. When your diet is centered around meat, vegetables become the side portions or options, as opposed to being the main feature. There are plenty of exotic and interesting vegetables and fruits, even local foods, which can be explored and added to meals. Dairy products, such as milk, eggs, and butter, can be easily substituted by non-dairy products that are coconut or almond-based. Tempeh and miso, fermented soy, as well as firm tofu, are often used instead of eggs or meat products in vegan meals.

Why Is Vegan Diet Healthy?

It is lower in calories, trans, and saturated fats (found in animal products), and plant-based foods are less processed and tend to be more natural than dairy and meat. As with any diet, there are advantages and disadvantages to the vegan diet, which will be explored later in this book. Overall, vegan or plant-based eating is sustainable and healthy, as long as you meet all of your dietary and nutrient requirements. A vegan diet is best to begin in stages, first by eliminating some meats (usually red meats), followed by poultry, fish, eggs, and dairy. Vegetarian is a good option for some people who wish to keep dairy and eggs in their diet either in the short term or long term. It can be a "gateway" to veganism from a meat-centric diet. The pace and mean by which you progress from your current way of eating to a plant-based diet should be an individual plan that fits within your lifestyle, taking into consideration any medical or health needs.

The different stages of vegetarianism are divided into the following categories:

Semi-vegetarian: This is not actually vegetarian, though it limits the types of meat in your diet. Most people who follow this way of eating eliminate or strictly limit red meats, such as beef and pork, eating mostly poultry and seafood. This diet usually includes eggs and dairy.

Pescatarian: the only meat consumed in this diet is fish, which is a step further from semi-vegetarian. Some people choose this diet in the long term, and they even incorporate the pescatarian diet with keto, as fish contains a lot of healthy fats and protein beneficial in a low-carb diet. This way of eating can also bridge a transition to veganism.

Lacto-vegetarian: This form of vegetarianism restricts all meat and egg products, although it includes dairy. Yogurt, cheese, milk, and butter are usually a part of this diet.

Ovo-vegetarian: Eggs are the only animal products included in this diet.

Lacto-ovo Vegetarian: As the name suggests, this combines the lacto and ovo types of vegetarian diet, which includes all dairy products and eggs while omitting all meat products.

While many people follow different variations of the vegetarian diet, sometimes, in combination with a low-carb diet or ketogenic diet, it can be either a long-term goal or a way to become more accommodated to a diet that is less reliant on meat products and processed food. In many variations of the keto diet, high levels of fats are often sourced from meats and dairy, which can still provide all of the benefits of keto eating. If you choose to incorporate both keto and vegan diets together, begin by reducing the number of animal products and decide which level you prefer (either one of the above vegetarian diets or progress to vegan).

Veganism: This form of vegetarianism differs from all other options for one reason—it is completely animal-free and plant-based. While it may take time to become comfortable with avoiding meat products, it is a process that should be done gently and carefully to ensure there are no nutrient deficiencies. It is the first goal of adapting to a vegan keto diet before reducing carbs and adding healthy, vegan fats to adjust for a long-term way of healthy eating and lifestyle.

Chapter 3: The Vegan Keto Diet: Why Is it the Most Beneficial Way to Eat?

The vegan and ketogenic diets both provide a lot of benefits on their own, and in combination, the impact on your health and weight loss are tremendous. On their own, both diets have specific characteristics, as indicated in the following chart. While both diets may seem completely opposite, they are both balanced and sustainable ways of eating:

Characteristics of the Keto Diet	Characteristics of the Vegan Diet
Low in carbohydrates and sugars	Plant-based. No animal products or by-products
Whole foods, as much as possible. Processed and packaged food items are avoided. Meat and dairy are included.	Whole foods, as much as possible. Processed and packaged food items are avoided.
Promotes the body's ability to switch from burning glucose and carbs to stored fats, resulting in weight loss	Vegan foods tend to be lower in calories and trans fats, making them easier to digest and metabolize

How does combining both vegan and ketogenic diet help you optimize your health and help you lose weight? When you factor in the low-carb intake of the keto diet, plus the high fiber and moderate-to-low caloric volume of plant-based foods, it draws the best of both diets into one powerful eating lifestyle. One of the major ways in which the ketogenic diet is successful in promoting a state of ketosis, which effectively produces ketones in your body to further break down fat instead of glucose as the primary source of fuel.

Vegan Ketosis: How Does Ketosis Work While on a Vegan Diet?

Achieving ketosis while on the vegan keto diet is like the regular ketogenic plan, only without the meat products. How is vegan ketosis different? First, as with regular keto, you'll need to increase your intake of healthy fats while eliminating sugar and carbs, as much as possible. A lot of fats can be found in animal products, and these are often used to increase fat content (eggs, milk, meat, oils), which can make it a challenge to find vegan alternatives. By nature, most meat alternatives are lower in fats and, therefore, do not produce as much energy for the fat-adapted body. This can be easily remedied with a bit of research and finding quality stores with the right food products. Coconut oil, seeds (hemp hearts, flaxseeds), nuts (specifically macadamia nuts), MCT oil, olive oil, avocados, and avocado oil are among the top choices for vegan fats. They are excellent sources of fatty acids and omega 3, and they can supplement your fuel, where plant-based options may seem limited.

Vegan Ketosis: How Is it Different From Regular Ketosis?

Ketosis is basically the same, whether you follow a regular ketogenic diet (including meat and dairy products) or a vegan keto plan. There may be some differences in the initial stages of ketosis, such as experiencing the keto "flu," which is characterized by temporary symptoms of fatigue, loss of focus and energy, and sometimes, nausea within the first two weeks. If your body is already adapted to a vegan diet, and you are strictly on this diet, these initial symptoms may manifest less and can be avoidable. This is because of the way plant-based foods are easily digested and your body may already be adapted to less carbohydrates, especially if you avoid processed foods (including packaged vegan foods). The major difference of regular ketosis versus vegan ketosis is in the level of fat you need to consume to reach and maintain the production of ketones, although overall, the experience and results are essentially the same.

The Advantages and Disadvantages of the Vegan Keto Diet

As with any diet, there are always considerations to make, concerning present health, life circumstances, and medical conditions. If you are experiencing a lot of stress or a major life event, it's best to make a slow transition or postpone any major dietary changes, even improvements. A diet that benefits your body includes your mind and well-being, and all components of your life should be weighed carefully. Generally, the vegan keto diet is beneficial for many reasons, and there are some characteristics or traits that may be considered less desirable or disadvantageous, depending on your expectations.

Advantages of the Vegan Keto Diet	Disadvantages of the Vegan Keto Diet
Diminishes the probability of developing certain types cancer, diabetes (type 2), and heart disease	Limits the amount of healthy fats due to no inclusion of meat, eggs, or dairy
Significantly lowers your chances of developing high blood pressure and related conditions	Plant-based fats are available, though may be expensive or hard to find in some regions or stores, depending on where you live.

Reduction of "bad" LDL cholesterol and improving good cholesterol	It requires effort to track and include all daily nutrients to ensure you are not deficient. Nutrient deficiencies can be avoided on a vegan keto diet, though it can easily occur when specific nutrients are missing (vitamin D, B12, for example).
Significant weight loss and higher levels of energy and mood stability	Lack of fresh, natural plant-based foods in some regions can make this diet challenging to follow.

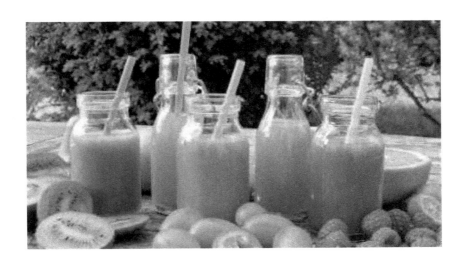

Chapter 4: Getting Started on the Vegan Keto Diet: Is it Right for You?

How do you know if the vegan keto lifestyle is for you? There are many factors to consider before you begin to ensure this way of eating is right for you. These include medical conditions, your lifestyle, dietary restrictions, and goals, as well as your commitment to achieving good health and weight loss. Considering how you eat currently is a good first step in determining how to proceed. For example, if you already adhere to a vegetarian or vegan diet, it will be much easier to gradually reduce carbohydrates in your diet until you reach the ketogenic level of up to 20 grams of carbs per day. On the other hand, if you are already following a ketogenic diet and looking to eliminate meat and dairy products, this will be a gradual process of eliminating one or several animal foods at a time until your diet is plant-based, while you keep a low-carb intake.

Before You Begin the Vegan Keto Diet: Steps to Take

What are the first steps? This depends on the status of your current diet and lifestyle and how well you can adjust and adapt to a new way of eating. While it is best to consult a medical professional about the impact of changing your diet on any specific health conditions, switching to a vegan keto diet is one of the best investments in your health for prevention against disease and improving health overall:

Step 1: How do you eat currently? Does your meal plan consist of careful planning, preparation, and budgeting, or do you often eat "on the go" with little time for consideration? If you have a busy life, simple and easy meals that can be prepared quickly or the night before are best for you. Keep this in mind when choosing recipes compatible with plant-based keto meals. Find some time to prepare meals for the week when it's convenient, such as on a Sunday evening before a workweek or another suitable time. Meal planning for a week will reduce a lot of stress and effort during busier days when there more things to juggle and coordinate.

Step 2: What does your grocery list look like? Do you stick with a list or buy compulsively? Buying impulsively or sporadically is fun sometimes, especially when you want to try a new recipe or food choice, though most, if not all, shopping is best planned with a list. This will keep you on track with cost, time, and making good food decisions. Examine your current list, if you have one: are most of the foods plant-based, low-carb, fresh, or processed and packaged? Is the list a combination of different foods or fairly rigid, centering around a limited number of foods or products?

Step 3: Where do you shop? Local and organic produce and food is the best option, though not always affordable or available, depending on where you live. If you have the option of shopping for local produce at farmer's markets and small, family-owned businesses, this will only support the local economy, and it will likely help your budget and improve the quality of food you eat. For baking supplies, try shopping in bulk or at stores that offer bulk as an option, as this will minimize packaging and keep portions and costs related to your food plan appropriate and relevant.

Step 4: What should be on your list? Once you decide that the vegan diet is right for you, it's time to work on a shopping list! When you review the list of foods appropriate for both ketogenic and vegan eating, you can search for effective alternatives to some (or all) of your foods to find out where they can be purchased, the costs, and when they are in season.

The First Week of Your Vegan Keto Diet

If you are planning on major results, this is one of the best ways to eat. Starting gradually by replacing one or two major items per week until your weekly grocery list is keto and plant-based is highly doable. Or, you can begin an overhaul with a fresh new list of vegan and keto-friendly foods. The second option may feel like more of a shock, and this may work for some people looking for drastic results within a relatively short period of time. The best approach for diving into this diet is a two-step process: adapting to plant-based eating and then reducing carbs.

Adapting to a Plant-Based Diet

Going vegan is a big change, especially if you enjoy meat, eggs, and dairy as a part of your diet. Replacing animal products with plant-based alternatives can be done gradually or quickly, depending on what pace works best for you. For example, start by eliminating red meats from your diet (pork, beef, etc.), and either replace them with poultry and fish or with a vegetarian substitute. Try this for one to two weeks before replacing all meat, including seafood and poultry, with plant-based options. At this stage, don't worry about lowering carbs, though you can try choosing soy and plant-based burgers and meat alternatives, instead of increasing the portion of rice, bread, or pasta you may currently enjoy. When in doubt, substitute a meat item with a vegetable option.

As you become adjusted to a meat-free diet, begin substituting the milk, yogurt, butter, and cheese items next. This may be as easy as cutting them out altogether or looking for a plant-based product. If you opt for a vegan cheese or butter substitute, read the ingredients carefully because even soy or vegetable alternatives can be loaded with extra salt, hidden sugars, and additives. Coconut oil and olive oil are excellent choices for baking and cooking instead of butter or margarine. Cultured yogurt, unsweetened, can replace the dairy version. Instead of flavoring food with cheese, try different herbs, spices, and grilled vegetables. This can work wonders for vegetarian burgers and casseroles.

It may take a while to switch your meat and dairy foods for vegan options, and for this reason, give yourself time. Changing too quickly may trigger cravings and switching back and forth or "cheating" on your diet. Plan ahead, take it slow, and try a new plant-based food before deciding whether to include them in your diet. If tofu or soy products sound unappealing to you, consider the various forms and ways soy can be prepared and enjoyed. Smoked tofu, pan-seared curried tempeh, and miso soup are all delicious variations that may change your outlook on soy foods and their limitless possibilities.

Going Vegan: Reducing Carbohydrates

Once a plant-based plan is established and you become comfortable with a regular plan, it's time to focus on reducing carbohydrates. Review your current shopping list or items you enjoy as part of a plant-based diet and determine the following:

- Do you include a lot of packaged and processed vegan foods in your diet? This may include energy bars, powders, dried fruit, and salty snacks.

- Check the sugar and glucose ingredients and levels in your diet. This includes fruits, preservatives (jams, condiments, etc.), and both natural and artificial sweeteners.
- Bread, pasta, grains, and rice: are these items included in your weekly shopping?
- Do you snack often and does this include chips, candies, and soft drinks?

All these items above are high in carbohydrates and should be either eliminated or strictly reduced. This can be done over a comfortable pace so that your body becomes used to smaller changes, instead of a complete overnight overhaul. Here are a few examples that will help get you started:

- Switch a bag of chips for almonds, walnuts, or peanuts. If you have a nut allergy, try dried coconut or fresh berries as a snack
- Replace soda, fruit juice, and other sugary drinks with regular water, sparkling water, or naturally unsweetened iced tea. Coffee is acceptable, without any added sugar, flavors, or preservatives. In some grocery stores, natural sodas with low or zero carb sweeteners are available and taste just like regular soda.
- One of the most challenging aspects of the keto diet is avoiding pasta and bread products. Baked goods are a staple in many diets. Grains and beans are also the main

sources of nutrients in many diets and also high in carbohydrates. Instead of getting rid of all of these items at once, work on reducing or removing one item at a time. There are vegan keto baked goods that can be easily prepared with simple ingredients. Vegetables and salads can take the place of grains, rice, and pasta.

- Take an inventory of the fresh and frozen fruits and vegetables in your diet. Begin to reduce carbs in this area by eliminating high-starch (and high-glucose) foods first, such as potatoes, peas, carrots, and bananas. Add or increase dark green vegetables, green beans, turnips, green peppers, berries, avocados, and coconut milk (unsweetened). Occasionally, small amounts of citrus fruit and rhubarb are acceptable.

It will take time to adjust your diet, and the results will be worth it. One of the greatest advantages of adapting to a vegan keto diet is the amount of knowledge you gain from learning about the nutritious value of foods. This experience will help encourage better and more thoughtful choices during your trips to the grocery store or local market.

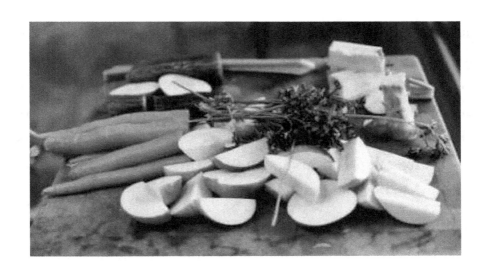

Chapter 5: What Foods Can You Eat on the Vegan Keto Diet?

Choosing Low-Carb, Plant-Based Foods to Meet Your Diet goals

Choosing the right vegan and ketogenic foods and keeping those choices consistent are the keys to success on this diet. Keep foods as natural and simple as possible, and build your diet and shopping list around these items.

Soy

Tofu, tempeh, and miso are all forms of soy. If you have an allergic reaction to soybeans and soy products, it may be beneficial to switch to fermented soy foods, such as miso and tempeh, which are usually more tolerable. Soy is considered a "superfood," as it contains most, if not all, required daily nutrients: protein, fiber, calcium, and vitamins. Some soy products are fortified with vitamin D and other nutrients. Fermented soy products contain B12, which is usually considered exclusive to meat and some dairy products.

One of the most versatile foods and a staple in many countries and regions around the world, soy can be incorporated into any meal of the day, including dessert and snacks. Complete meals and food preparation techniques are centered around soy, which makes it a primary source of a vegan diet. Some prepared soy products may contain additives and marinades with sweeteners that contribute to an increase in carbohydrates. The best option for soy is natural, unsweetened, and unflavored tofu and tempeh products. This includes soy milk, yogurts, and other soy or dairy substitutes. Avoid any items with added flavors (natural or unnatural), as they will increase glucose levels.

Seeds and Nuts

Almonds, walnuts, pumpkin seeds, peanuts, flaxseeds, and hemp hearts are all low in carb content and highly nutritious options for a vegan keto diet. Pumpkin seeds are high in protein, magnesium, iron, and zinc. Just a handful a day as a snack can provide a significant amount of your daily needs. Hemp seeds contain healthy fats that work well to increase the overall amount of fats you need to maintain ketosis. These seeds also contain protein and have been known to reduce blood pressure and provide energy. Sunflower seeds contain amino acids and protein, similar to pumpkin seeds; they can be added as a snack to your diet in between meals.

Chia Seeds

These amazing seeds deserve a category of their own because of its numerous benefits and usability in many meals, drinks, and supplements. Originating from South America, chia seeds are high in protein, amino acids, fiber, and vitamins. They have grown in popularity in many diets, including paleo, ketogenic, and vegan diets. Smoothies, baked goods, salads, and desserts are just a few options where chia seeds can be added. Mixed with other forms of protein such as seeds or soy to create puddings and smoothies or as a topping to a salad or main meal, chia seeds are easy to find and available in most grocery stores. They are usually found in bulk stores, where they are less expensive and may be available in several varieties.

Mushrooms

Shiitake, portobello, and other varieties of mushrooms can be enjoyed on a vegan keto diet.

Dark, Green Leafy Vegetables

One of the best features of the vegan keto diet is the number of vegetable options that are low in carbohydrates. When considering all low-carb options, green leafy vegetables are the most beneficial. These include kale, spinach, and arugula. Parsley, cilantro, dill, and many others can fit this category as well. Don't let the bitterness and unfamiliarity of kale deter you from trying them. There are plenty of recipes that enhance and change the flavor of these dark greens with various spices and oils. A simple example is baked kale chips, which are easy to prepare with a few ingredients. This is featured in the recipe section of this book. Spinach is a great addition to tofu scramble, skillet meals, and salads.

Cruciferous Vegetables: Cauliflower and Broccoli

These vegetables include cauliflower and broccoli, both of which are high in fiber.

Zucchini

This vegetable gets a special mention because it can be altered to replace some high-carb ingredients found in pasta dishes. Sliced, thin zucchini can make a great "noodle" for a lasagne, while spiral-sliced zucchini can replace noodles in soups or spaghetti or as a way to dress up a salad.

Fruits: Avocados, Berries, and on Occasion, Citrus Fruits

In the order that they are listed, enjoy avocado often; enjoy berries sometimes and citrus fruits on occasion. Avocado contains the least amount of carbohydrates of all fruits and can be enjoyed daily, as the carb content is very low. Berries have a low glycaemic level and can be added in small amounts to coconut milk as a treat or on their own as a snack. All berries are included: blackberries, strawberries, raspberries, and blueberries. Citrus fruits are more moderate in carbs, although they can be enjoyed in small doses. A splash of freshly squeezed lemon or lime in carbonated water or any recipe would be good. Rhubarb, though not often available and seasonal, is another low-to-moderate carb fruit that can be enjoyed in moderation.

Avocado

In addition to listing avocado with the fruit options, it is a valuable source of nutrients that can play a major role in your diet.

MCT and Coconut Oil

Coconut oil is readily available in most food stores, and MCT oil, the fat extract of coconut oil, is an excellent way to supplement the healthy fats in a vegan keto diet.

Low-Carb Sweeteners

These may seem too good to be real, as they taste like sugar while remaining completely carb-free or low-carb. Monk fruit is the best option and the most sugar-like in taste and texture. Other options include stevia and erythritol. Xylitol is another low-carb sweetener, though can be dangerous for pets, and should be avoided if you have a pet. Overall, all low-carb sweeteners are safe and can be found combined for maximum sweetness and taste.

Fermented Food Options

Tempeh and miso are fermented soy options, and other fermented foods are similarly keto and vegan-friendly, with many nutrients. Sauerkraut and kimchi are two main options that can be added as a side dish or snack. They both have a strong flavor and may be considered an acquired taste, though they can be enjoyed in small portions, along with a curried tofu dish or as a side with a soup or salad.

Seaweed and Sea Vegetables

Kelp, seaweed, and other sea-based vegetables are an excellent source of calcium, protein, and fiber. Seaweed is the most popular, usually found in sushi dishes. It can also be enjoyed as a ready-made snack in dried form.

How to Choose Foods and Balance Your Nutritional Needs

When you create your first shopping list, keep in mind your nutritional needs. For example, if you are active and want to build muscle by weight training, increasing the variety and level of protein could be a specific goal to keep in mind when choosing food. Maintain a regular metabolism, which means adding lots of fresh foods, natural produce, and a lot of fiber as major components of your diet.

Vegan Keto Bread: How to Make it and Add Into Your Regular Meals

Traditionally, baked goods, such as bread, pastries, and cakes are full of sugar and carbohydrates, which automatically eliminates them as options for a vegan keto diet. Fortunately, there are alternative ingredients that can be creatively used to recreate vegan and ketogenic versions of many baked foods to satisfy your craving. Before you consider baking the vegan keto way, create a simple and practical pantry of plant-based and ketogenic ingredients for your baking creations:

- **Low-carb sweeteners**. Monk fruit, stevia, and various other low-carb sweeteners can be found in dried granules like sugar and kept in a sealed container for a long time.

- **Almond and coconut flour**. Almond flour tends to be more costly and can often be combined with coconut flour in many recipes. It's also available in bulk. Coconut flour is drier and combines well with almond. Both options are best to have on hand, as they can be used separately or together in a variety of recipes.
- **Baking powder and baking soda**
- **Psyllium husk powder**
- **Vinegar**. Depending on the varieties of foods you enjoy and the recipes you create, vinegar tends to be low in carb content and can be safely added to many dishes
- **Oil**. Olive, avocado, and coconut oil are the best options
- **Nut butter**. Almond and peanut butter are the most popular options. Sesame seed butter is sometimes overlooked, although it's a protein-rich option that can easily replace other types of nut butter. Hazelnut butter is another option.
- **Coconut milk and cream**. These are invaluable ingredients for many dishes, from cakes to curries and puddings. They are available in cartons or cans.
- **Nutritional yeast**. This is good if you plan on baking vegan keto bread.
- **Psyllium husk** is a good ingredient to have, as it can effectively replace gluten in baking. It's good for your metabolism, high in fiber, and helps thicken or act as a

"glue" that keeps baked goods together. Psyllium can be bought in powder form and sometimes available in bulk, usually in natural food stores (or online).

- **Flaxseeds, chia seeds, and hemp hearts**. These may be optional or integral ingredients in a lot of recipes and a good boost of nutrients with any meal.

These ingredients create a strong foundation for many basic vegan keto baking recipes, which can be further expanded to include extracts, seeds, dried coconut flakes, and other low-carb options. There are many powders and supplements available in the market, specifically in natural and bulk foods stores. However, it's best to read the ingredients thoroughly to rule out additive and other items that add glucose or carbs. Keep ingredients as natural and as simple as possible. One brand of coconut flour should be the same as another, though watch for unusual or too many ingredients. Coconut milk can be sweetened or enhanced with additives, and for this reason, only unsweetened, pure versions of this milk should be included.

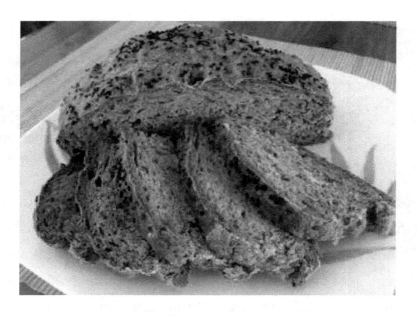

Vegan Keto Bread Recipe

Creating a vegan keto bread is not as difficult as it seems, though it may require a few "practice runs" to find the right recipe for your taste. Some breads can either be too hard or crumbly, and others lack the texture. In this section, three bread recipes are provided with their unique characteristics and flavors.

Flour-Free Almond Bread

This is a simple recipe that can be a good way to get acquainted with keto (and vegan) baking. It is best to begin with an easy recipe that doesn't require too much preparation or too many ingredients. This bread requires just three basic ingredients. It's gluten-free and can be supplemented with a dash of flaxseeds or hemp hearts for an additional boost of nutrients. Salt is also another option, depending on your preference. The main ingredients are as follows.

- 2 teaspoons psyllium husk powder
- 2 teaspoons of baking powder
- Olive or coconut oil (1-2 teaspoons)
- 1 ½ cups almond meal
- ½ cup of water

You need to add optional ingredients, as well as water, to make this recipe work. Almond meal is used instead of almond flour, as the almond meal retains the outer skin or shell of the almonds, while the flour doesn't (the skins are needed in this recipe). Keep some extra water on hand, just in case the dough needs a bit more. The water, when combined with the psyllium husk powder, will create a gel consistency, creating an effective egg replacement. Preheat the oven to 350 degrees. Spray some coconut oil or olive oil on a baking sheet and set aside. Mix the almond meal and baking powder in a medium-sized bowl. Combine the psyllium husk powder and water in another bowl, smaller in size. Stir the mixture for approximately 8 minutes to make a gel. Combine with the almond meal and baking powder and whisk all ingredients until thoroughly blended. Divide the mixture into 7-8 small muffin-like patties and bake in the oven for 25 minutes. For an easier bake, these can be prepared in a muffin sheet or shaped by hand and baked. Serve warm or cold. These can be toasted and used like regular bread.

Vegan Keto Seed Bread

This bread contains nuts and seeds and holds well together, unlike a lot of bread recipes that do not contain eggs. Psyllium husk powder is a good egg replacement, and for this reason, consider using this option with all bread and baking recipes where eggs would normally be used. There are considerably more ingredients in this bread than the first recipe, though the amounts are small and can be easily found and combined.

- 1 cup of water
- ½ cup hazelnuts
- ½ cup slivered or raw almonds
- ½ cup sesame seeds
- ½ cup pumpkin seeds
- ½ cup sunflower seeds
- ¼ cup chia seeds (any variety)
- 3 tablespoons olive or coconut oil
- 1 teaspoon sea salt
- 2 tablespoons psyllium husk powder

Preheat the oven to 360 degrees and prepare and measure all of the ingredients. Combine all ingredients, except for the water and psyllium husk, into a blender or food processor and blend until all are evenly ground. Add the water and psyllium husk powder and continue to mix. Prepare a small, rectangular baking dish by lining or coating with coconut or olive oil and pour the mixture evenly. Bake for 55-60 minutes. Keep an eye on the oven during the last ten minutes to ensure that it is baking thoroughly. Allow the bread to cool slightly before slicing to serve.

This recipe can be modified by increasing the amount of some nuts and seeds to replace others. For example, if you do not want to include sunflower seeds, substitute by doubling almonds or pumpkin seeds or another item. Enhance the particular flavor (nuts and seeds) by doubling the portion of some and reducing one or two of the other options.

Simple Vegan Keto Bread

This recipe is simple, although it includes a few additional ingredients compared to the first option, and it has fewer nuts and seeds (a few can be added as an option if desired). This recipe includes two different types of flour: coconut and almond. These work well together with their texture for many recipes, including crepes and cakes. Guar gum is also used in this recipe, along with psyllium husk, as a way to thicken the dough.

- 1 cup of almond flour
- 1/8 cup of coconut flour
- 1/8 cup of ground linseed

- 5-6 tablespoons of water
- ¼ cup psyllium husk powder
- 1 tablespoon guar gum
- 1 tablespoon baking powder
- 1 teaspoon sea salt
- Dash of spices (sage, oregano, rosemary, etc.)
- 1/8 cup coconut oil
- 1 tablespoon apple cider vinegar
- 1 cup of water (separate from the 5-6 tablespoons mentioned above)

Preheat the oven to 400 degrees. Combine all of the dry ingredients, with the exception of the linseed, and mix everything in a medium bowl. In a separate bowl, combine the linseed and water (5-6 tablespoons) and set aside. After 10 minutes, check the thickness of the linseed mixture to ensure that it has thickened, and add it to the remaining dry ingredients. Add 1 cup of water and the apple cider vinegar. Continue to mix all ingredients and knead into a dough. Form small buns or loaves on a prepared baking sheet, coated in olive or coconut oil, and bake for 50-60 minutes. Check the progress between 50-60 minutes, and bake the bread for an extra 10-15 minutes after 60, if needed. Serve warm or cool. These can be sliced and toasted.

Adding Vegan Keto Bread to Your Regular Meals

Vegan keto bread can easily fit into any meal of the day or as a light snack, toasted with nut butter, vegan butter, or cream cheese. A bread with a more seedy, hearty texture will work well with soups and salads, and lighter breads make an excellent choice for breakfast. Light to medium bread buns work well with vegan burgers, and a lighter, thinner crepe-like wrap can also be good with breakfast or wraps (included in the breakfast recipes). In general, vegan keto bread can take the place of their carb-heavy versions. If one or two recipes are too heavy or unappealing, there are many other variations and recipes to consider. It's an opportunity to become acquainted with the "anatomy" of what makes a good bread to your taste, and experimenting with as many options as possible will provide a lot of choices, more than with regular bread!

Tools and Equipment for a Vegan Keto Diet

There are many gadgets, innovative kitchen appliances, and state-of-the-art blenders and juicers that can create anything imaginable. Fortunately, for the vegan keto diet, these can be helpful, though not completely necessary. Simple, easy-to-use tools and a good blender or food processor can take care of many recipes. Here are some standard, basic items to have when creating recipes:

- **A blender and food processor**. A handheld blender (or small, cup-sized) is a good idea for making quick, single-serve smoothies or milkshakes. A food processor is ideal for crushing nuts and seeds and combining ingredients (both wet and dry) for all your recipes.
- **Whisk**. This is a simple, handheld tool useful for mixing ingredients by hand.
- **Skillet (one medium, one large)**. Having at least two cast-iron skillets are great for stir fry dishes and making breakfast crepes or tofu scramble. Cast iron skillets are heated on low to medium heat (never above medium) with coconut, olive, or avocado oil before frying or sautéing meals.
- **Spatulas, large ladle, and forks**. Spatulas are used in mixing, flipping, and turning over foods while cooking. A strong wooden or stainless-steel spoon is good for stirring.
- **Glass or durable (reusable and resealable) plastic containers** to store, freeze, and refrigerate prepared foods and ingredients
- **Glass jars** for spices, herbs, teas, and other dry ingredients in your pantry

- **One or two strong, durable graters (one fine and one for larger pieces)** is ideal for shredding vegetables for patties, hash browns, and salads. Two graters, one of each size, is recommended to accommodate most recipes.
- **Stainless steel cooking pots (one medium and one large)** for soups and stews and making curries and similar sauces
- **Measuring utensils**, such as cups, teaspoons, and tablespoons are helpful in ensuring that all ingredients are measured accurately.
- **A good quality set of knives and a sharpener** for slicing vegetables, fruits, and baked goods

There are many other items that can be added, though these utensils, tools, and equipment are a good foundation for most recipes.

Special & Unique Ingredients to Consider for the Diet

If you are adventurous when it comes to trying new foods, spices, and meals from other cultures and regions, here are some tips to keep in mind to avoid adding unwanted carbs, meat products, or both. If you shop in a store that specializes in various Asian foods, you'll notice a lot of noodles and rice and starch-rich products, which should be avoided. Fortunately, there are a lot of keto and vegan-friendly options that make it easy, such as soy products (tofu, soy milk, and miso), fermented foods (kimchi cabbage and radishes are popular), and lots of greens. If you are having difficulty finding vegan keto-friendly foods at your local grocery store, look for a large or medium-sized Asian grocery store, which can offer many more options.

Bakeries and coffee shops offer a lot of sugary and carb-heavy foods, which should be eliminated, though some specialty bakeries are popping up in some cities that specialize in ketogenic, vegan, and gluten-free goods. These are worth checking out to find out which ingredients are used in their foods. Shops that specialize in food products that cater to specific dietary needs are often very willing to provide as much information possible to assure their customers that their foods have good in quality. Quality ingredients are the most important and should be reviewed before making final decisions on purchasing from one of these stores. Reading reviews and feedback is another good idea.

Delicatessens, local farmers markets, and grocers with fresh street-side produce are the best options, as they usually provide fresh and local goods. Delicatessens tend to feature meat, cheese, and dairy, though some may offer vegan alternatives as well.

Chapter 6: Frequently Asked Questions and Answers About the Vegan Keto Diet

How Does the Vegan Keto Diet Maximize Weight Loss?

Going both vegan and keto gives you the best of both diets. A plant-based diet is lower in trans and saturated fats and higher in healthier fats, which is better for your overall health. A vegan diet is also higher in fiber since it is entirely based on vegetation, which keeps metabolism regular and weight manageable. The ketogenic diet, on the other hand, reduces the amount of carbohydrates while increasing healthy fats and maintaining protein. This not only keeps your body healthy and strong, but it also increases fat burning through ketosis (described in chapter 1). While sticking with the plant-based foods and adapting to ketogenic eating at the same time, all of the benefits from both diets are combined to provide all the benefits to maximize weight loss and keep your weigh at a consistent level once your goal is achieved.

Will I Meet All of My Daily Nutritional Requirements?

It is important that all your daily requirements for nutrients are met in order to avoid developing deficiencies. Some of the most common deficiencies are vitamin D and B12, especially on a vegan diet, as dairy and meat contain one or both (many milk products are fortified with vitamin D). Other minerals and vitamins that can be challenging to get from a vegan diet are iron, protein, calcium, and magnesium. Fortunately, a lot of soy products and non-dairy, vegan milks contain vitamin D and B12. Dark green vegetables are among the best sources for minerals, including iron, which is often low in vegan diets. Keeping track of the foods you eat and the nutritional value for each are important in maintaining a balanced diet.

Is it an Easy Diet to Follow?

There are challenges to following a vegan keto diet, though there are ways to make it easier to adapt and to follow. One thought to keep in mind when shopping is that every regular food item has a vegan keto alternative. For butter, there is a nut butter, vegan butter, or oil as an alternative. For sugar, there are low-carb sweeteners, and in place of dairy, there are coconut and soy-based options. The list and availability of both keto and vegan foods is continually growing and improving over time. It's beneficial to research as much as possible about natural supplements and vitamins while avoiding synthetic and processed versions, which can appear similar to their natural counterparts.

What Happens if I "Cheat" by Eating Animal-Based or High-Carb Food?

This will occur from time to time, either by accident or when there is a special meal or occasion where vegan keto food options are not readily available. Sometimes, it can be impossible to plan ahead for special dietary requests. This can occur when you are on vacation or in an unfamiliar region with a completely different assortment of fruits and vegetables. In these situations, it's best to stick with vegan first, as much as possible. And then, avoid carbs when they are obvious, and simply do not worry about reducing carbs until after the occasion. Remember that this is a temporary situation, not a setback or a failure. Everyone can take a break or "carb up" (increase carbohydrate intake) for a variety of reasons, such as vigorous exercise, hiking, cycling, marathons, etc. There is always another opportunity to jump back into vegan keto.

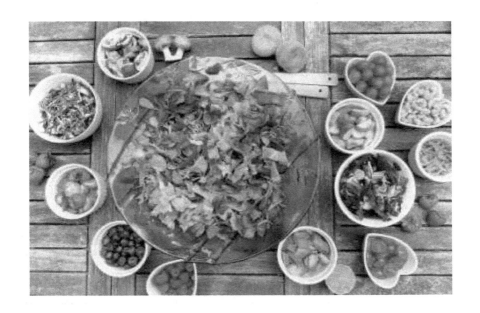

Chapter 7: Meal Planning and Preparation

The essential food items you need to start the diet and prepare for meal planning include a 4-week vegan keto masterplan.

Meal planning and preparation are the most important part of following and sticking to a healthy vegan keto diet. This plan is a guide to get you started on meal choices, with all of the corresponding recipes listed in the following chapter, under various meals of the day. To keep the plan easier to follow, just breakfast, lunch, and dinner are listed. Vegan keto snacks and desserts, while they are significantly good, should not be eaten in excess. The main focus is on the three main meals of the day.

First Week: Keeping it Simple

Week 1	Su	M	T	W	T	F	Sa
Breakfast	Avocado Coconut power smoothie	Tofu scramble	Curried Tofu scramble	Fruit and Coconut yogurt cup	Tofu scramble	Curried Tofu scramble	Vegan Keto breakfast bagels
Lunch	Avocado and tofu bake	Avocado Toast	Mediterranean sandwich	Avocado Toast	Sesame tofu bake	Peanut butter and toast	Eggplant with vegan cheese
Dinner	Butternut squash soup	Broccoli and cauliflower rice	Zucchini noodle pasta	Butternut squash baked with smoked tofu	Curried pumpkin soup	Vegan Keto platter	Vegan keto chili

Second Week: Adding More Options

Week 2	Su	M	T	W	T	F	S
Breakfast	Avocado Coconut power smoothie	Tofu scramble	Vegan keto breakfast bagels	Fruit and Coconut yogurt cup	Tofu scramble	Curried Tofu scramble	Vegan Keto breakfast bagels
Lunch	Avocado and tofu bake	Curried cabbage	Pizza stuffed peppers	Tandoori tempeh	Fried mushrooms and Brussel sprouts		
Dinner	Vegan keto chili (leftover from Sat)	Cauliflower macaroni and cheese					

Third Week: Getting Creative

Week 3	Su	M	T	W	T	F	S
Breakfast	Skillet breakfast	Chia pudding	Curried Tofu scramble	Fruit and Coconut yogurt cup	Skillet breakfast	Vegan keto crepes	Shakshuka
Lunch	Avocado and tofu bake	Zucchini noodles and avocado sauce	Curried tempeh and snow peas	Avocado toast	Pizza stuffed peppers	Smoked tofu and arugula	Peanut butter and toast
Dinner	Skillet meal (choice of 1-11)						

Fourth Week: Staying on Track

Week 4	Su	M	T	W	T	F	S
Breakfast	Chia pudding	Avocado smoothie	Tofu scramble	Fruit and coconut yogurt cup	Tofu scramble	Curried Tofu scramble	Tofu and spinach pies
Lunch	Peanut butter and toast	Curried cabbage	Sesame tofu bake	Grilled "cheese"	Lettuce sandwich wrap	Tandoori tempeh	Curried broccoli and kale soup
Dinner	Vegan moussaka	Skillet meal (choice of 1-11)					Cauliflower macaroni and cheese

Vegan Keto Recipes

Breakfast

Tofu Scramble

Tofu is a superfood that can take the place of many types of meat and dairy products, including eggs, which are frequently used in breakfast meals. The consistency of tofu can vary from soft to firm, depending on the dish you create. Tofu takes on any flavor and is best marinated overnight or for a few hours to absorb spices, juices, or broth to combine the tastes together before cooking. To prepare this dish, soak one block of firm tofu in a container or bowl of vegetable broth, black pepper, and salt. The ingredients are simple, easy to find, and can be modified to add spice or different flavors:

- 2 cups of vegetable broth
- One block of firm tofu, or the equivalent
- 2 teaspoons of turmeric
- 1 teaspoon salt
- 1 teaspoon black pepper

Wash and soak the block of tofu in a bowl of vegetable broth so that it is fully immersed. Add a dash of salt and pepper and mix into the broth before marinating. Keep in a closed container and leave in the refrigerator overnight so that it is ready for breakfast in the morning. Heat the skillet on medium and add turmeric and a couple of tablespoons of vegetable broth from the marinated tofu. Drain the tofu and reserve ½ cup of liquid. Mash the tofu and add another teaspoon of turmeric, salt, and black pepper and mix well, then transfer the mashed tofu to the skillet and cook. The combination of broth and turmeric will give the tofu a golden appearance, similar to scrambled eggs. The tofu takes roughly 5-7 minutes to cook fully and can be enjoyed right away.

There are some tasty ingredients to consider for enhancing the flavor:

- Chili pepper or flakes
- Chopped or sliced green peppers and onions: a small portion of these can be fried into the tofu scramble
- Spinach (fresh or frozen)
- Fried mushrooms (any variety)

Curried Tofu Scramble

This dish is a variation on the regular version, which marinates the tofu in curry spice the night before, along with all the ingredients in the recipe above. Just like the regular tofu scramble, this spicier option can include the same vegetables above and a few others for consideration:

- Okra
- Red peppers
- Green beans

Add the following spices to the vegetable broth and tofu to marinate overnight. Drain the next morning and retain ½ cup for frying the tofu.

- Two tablespoons of curry powder or paste
- 1 teaspoon garlic powder or salt
- 2-3 bay leaves, crushed
- 1 teaspoon chili powder or flakes
- Black pepper and salt (just a dash or more, depending on your preference)
- ½ teaspoon garam masala (optional)
- 1 teaspoon turmeric
- 1 teaspoon cumin

Prepare in a skillet like the regular tofu scramble and serve with fresh coriander or parsley.

Avocado Coconut Power Smoothie

Smoothies are easy, healthy, and delicious any time of day, and especially a good option for breakfast. They provide a good dose of daily nutrients in a fraction of time it takes to prepare a full meal. As this is the first meal of the day, it's important to include a lot of nutrients and healthy fats, which both coconut and avocado provide. Only a few key ingredients are required for this quick smoothie:

- 1 medium or large ripe avocado
- 1 can of coconut (or the equivalent – roughly 1 ½ cups)
- ¼ cup coconut cream (unsweetened)
- 2 tablespoons monk fruit, swerve or stevia
- 2 tablespoons of collagen protein powder (vanilla flavor)

Combine the fleshy parts of the avocados, coconut milk, cream in a blender and mix until all of the ingredients are smooth. If the blend is not thick enough, add more coconut cream or half of another avocado to thicken the smoothie. Add the sweetener and collagen powder, then continue to mix until evenly combined and serve. Garnish with unsweetened coconut flakes, if desired.

If you want to add more protein to this recipe, add a dollop of sesame, almond, or peanut butter (unsweetened, no additives). Hemp and flaxseeds or oil is another good option. MCT or coconut oil will add more healthy fats to this smoothie. For a good boost of protein, healthy fats, and nutrients, feel free to add all of the above.

Vegan Keto Crepes

Enjoying crepes does not have to be a thing of the past because there is a low-carb alternative that is just as tasty, with some delicious toppings as well. Crepes, like pancakes, are prepared with whole wheat flour, which is replaced with almond and coconut flour, which has an easy consistency to work with for many vegan and keto baking recipes. This crepe recipe specifically can also be used as roti or wrap for stir fry and curries as a flatbread. Eggs can be replaced with coconut cream and flaxseeds:

- 2 tablespoons coconut cream mixed with flaxseeds (mix separately, preferably in a blender to combine well)
- ¾ cup almond milk
- ½ cup water
- 1 cup almond flour
- 1-2 tablespoons of monk fruit, stevia or a similar low-carb sweetener
- Olive or coconut oil for frying (as much as needed)

Heat the skillet on medium and mix the sweetener and almond flour in a large or medium bowl, whichever you prefer. Add into the bowl the flaxseed mix, coconut cream, water, and almond milk and continue to stir. Ensure all ingredients are combined equally and that the mixture is not too thick but light and slightly thicker than milk. Once the oil is heated, pour the equivalent of

½ cup of the mixture and fry for 2 minutes or until the crepe can be lifted easily (without breaking apart) with a spatula. Gently flip the crepe and cook the opposite side. Once you achieve a golden hue on both sides, transfer to a plate, add the topping of your choice, and fold.

- Whipped coconut cream (store-bought coconut whipping cream or made with a sweetener and ½ cup of cream in an electric blender)
- Cinnamon
- Fresh or lightly stewed berries and rhubarb
- Nut butter spread (almond, peanut or hazelnut butter)
- Cocoa powder sprinkled on the crepe or melted dark chocolate (unsweetened). Combine melted cocoa or chocolate with nut butter for another option
- Sliced avocado drizzled in coconut cream and sesame seeds
- Low-carb syrup

Almond flour is the most versatile and easy to use low-carb flour for vegan keto baking, though it can be expensive. Another option to consider is combining a ½ cup of coconut flour with ½ cup almond flour. Coconut flour is drier and more challenging to work with on its own, though it can be a good combination with almond and is less costly. Purchasing both flours in bulk is another option to keep within a budget and have enough to prepare a variety of recipes.

Fruit and Coconut Yogurt Cup

This delicious and quick breakfast can be prepared with all plant-based and natural ingredients without all the carbohydrates. While many fruits contain a lot of carbs, berries tend to rank low on this scale, which makes them acceptable as a tasty addition to many meals, either fresh or frozen. In this recipe, fresh, locally harvested berries work best. The cup can be mixed or layered, beginning with the fruit, then the yogurt, followed by toppings:

- 1 cup of coconut-cultured yogurt (plain or vanilla)
- ½ cup keto granola (see recipe later)
- 1 cup of fresh berries (blueberries, strawberries, raspberries, blackberries, or a combination of these)

In a tall glass or cup, add the fruit to the bottom, followed by a second layer of yogurt. Add the keto granola as a topping, and add these options:

- Dark, unsweetened cocoa or chocolate chips or shavings
- Shredded coconut or flakes (unsweetened)
- Flax and hemp seeds
- Crushed peanuts or almonds
- Cinnamon

For an additional fruit option, rhubarb is a low-carb fruit that is very sour in taste and which can be stewed and sweetened with monk fruit or another low-carb sweetener. Rhubarb compliments the sweetness of the berries as well for a good mix either below the yogurt or mixed together and garnished with the toppings of your choice.

To add more protein to this serving, soak ¼ cup of chia seeds in the yogurt for at least two hours or overnight, then use the thickened mixture to top the berries, or mix them together. The chocolate or coconut flakes can similarly be added to the yogurt and blended instead of a topping.

Vegan Keto Breakfast Bagels

Bagels are carb-heavy, as well as other baked bread and pastries, and a ketogenic, plant-based option can be substituted to satisfy this craving. In keto baking, wheat flour is typically switched to coconut and almond flour. Eggs, cheese, and butter are also typically used to prepare keto bagels and other baked goods, which can be simply replaced with plant-based alternatives, without compromising flavor:

- 1/3 cup of ground flaxseeds
- ½ cup of sesame butter
- ¼ cup psyllium powder or collagen powder (or both combined into ¼ cup)
- 1 tablespoon of water
- 1 tablespoon of baking powder
- Sesame seeds

Combine all the dry ingredients (flaxseeds, collagen or psyllium powder, and baking powder) in a medium bowl and mix well. The oven must be warmed to 380 degrees as you prepare the ingredients. In a separate bowl, whisk the water and sesame butter thoroughly, then add to the dry ingredients. Continue to mix with a spoon or by hand until it becomes a dough and can be kneaded. Prepare a baking tray and line with parchment paper. Form bagel-shaped molds by hand or by rolling into a 3" ball, gently flattening on the paper and cutting out a 1" hole in the center. Continue until all the mixture is used, which should make about 4-6 small, thin bagels. Bake the bagels for 45 minutes or when they have become slightly crispy and golden brown. Slice, toast, or enjoy fresh out of the oven with one of the following toppings:

- Avocado and vegan cheese
- Nut butter spread (peanut or hazelnut butter)
- Tomato, basil leaves, and avocado slices

To add more flavor inside the bagels and for a sweeter option, combine 2 tablespoons of low-carb sweetener and 1 teaspoon of cinnamon powder for cinnamon bagels. For "everything" bagels, combine poppy seeds, sesame seeds, dried garlic, and onion powder in a small bowl and add as a topping to the bagel shapes just before baking.

Chia Pudding (Vanilla)

Chia seeds are considered a "superfood" due to the many health benefits they provide as a part of a regular diet or meal plan. One of the most popular ways to enjoy them is by adding the seeds to a pudding recipe. They provide a good source of fiber, protein, and calcium, and help improve digestion, cardiovascular health, and weight loss. This chia pudding is a basic, vanilla recipe, though many flavors can be added to change the taste and texture:

- ½ cup of chia seeds (any variety)
- 1 teaspoon vanilla
- 1 cup of coconut milk
- 1-2 teaspoons cinnamon (optional topping)
- ¼ cup stevia, monk fruit or similar low-carb sweetener
- 1 cup of coconut cream (similar to the thickness in dairy full fat cream)

Combine the coconut milk, cream, and sweetener and whisk together gently in a medium bowl, then add the vanilla and chia seeds and continue to mix. Blend carefully to ensure all the chia seeds are evenly spaced in the mixture. Some of the seeds may stick to the utensils and sides of the bowl. If this occurs, gently slide them back into the mixture and stir until all ingredients are even. Move the liquid to a sealable container and refrigerate overnight and enjoy in the morning with a sprinkle of cinnamon on top of each serving.

The toppings and flavors for chia pudding options are limitless, and they provide a fun and healthy way to enjoy this highly nutritious treat.

- Add melted dark, unsweetened chocolate (approximately ¼ cup) to the ingredients for a chocolate or cocoa pudding
- Fresh berries can be added to the mix or as a topping. If frozen berries are available, blend with the coconut milk and cream mixture, before adding the chia seeds, sweetener, and vanilla
- Cardamom spice can be used in place of cinnamon
- A blend of or one of these nuts can make a delicious addition to the pudding, as a topping or mixed with the chia seeds: almonds, macadamia nuts, hazelnuts, peanuts, or walnuts
- Blend the coconut cream and milk with pumpkin puree (about ½ cup), then add the remaining ingredients in the original recipe. This variation can be topped with roasted pumpkin seeds
- Hemp hearts and MCT oil make excellent supplements to chia pudding

The advantage of this recipe is having different options and how simple it is to make. Chia pudding can be a regular breakfast option, a snack, or a meal substitute in situations where you need a quick, nutritious solution.

Shakshuka

This dish is popular in Middle Eastern cuisine. Traditionally, this dish is comprised of eggs poached in a spicy tomato sauce combined with vegetables and meat, peppers, and herbs, sometimes topped with cheese. For the ketogenic diet, this meal works perfectly, and it can easily be adapted to fit the vegan keto diet with a few modifications to the ingredients:

- firm tofu, half a block (cubed, 1 or 2-inches)
- 1 small can of tomatoes
- 1 bell pepper, diced
- ½ cup diced tomatoes (optional)
- 1 garlic clove, crushed
- 1 tablespoon chili pepper powder or flakes
- 1 tablespoon cumin seeds
- Dash of black pepper and salt (sea salt or pink Himalayan salt)
- Parsley for garnish
- 2-3 tablespoons of olive oil

Heat a skillet on low to medium heat and add 2-3 tablespoons of olive oil and all of the spices, herbs and cumin seeds. Fry for 2-3 minutes, then add garlic and bell pepper and continue to fry for 2-3 more minutes. Decrease the heat to low, and add the diced tomatoes and tomato sauce. Stir the ingredients into the sauce and let it stew for 10 minutes while preparing the tofu.

Note: Tofu can be marinated in tomato sauce or vegetable broth the night before to add flavor or simply use as is.

In a separate, small skillet, add one tablespoon of olive oil and coat the pan evenly. Heat on medium heat and add tofu cubes and increase heat to sear. Remove the skillet from the heat once the tofu is fully cooked and add the seared tofu to the spiced tomato sauce, carefully stirring in the pieces and coating them evenly with sauce.

Skillet Breakfast

Stir fry meals and skillet dishes are not just for lunch or dinner. Fresh peppers, mushrooms, and other vegetables can combine well in a skillet for an easy, healthy first meal of the day in a matter of minutes. If you enjoy a quick meal before you leave for work, cut the vegetables the night before and store in a container; airtight would be best. Leave it overnight in the fridge.

- 2 tablespoons sesame seeds
- 4-5 small or medium mushrooms, sliced
- 2-3 basil leaves
- 1 green pepper sliced lengthwise into strips
- 2 tablespoons of olive oil
- Smoked tofu or tempeh (half a block or package)
- 2 stalks of celery, diced into small 1" pieces

Heat the skillet and add olive oil for approximately one minute on a medium level. Add celery first, followed by tofu or tempeh, then green peppers, and basil leaves. Leave mushrooms to add once most of the vegetables and tofu are nearly cooked yet crunchy, and continue to sauté it on low to medium heat. Sprinkle sesame seeds on top and gently mix into the ingredients before serving.

If you like a spicy version of this dish, add chili peppers or flakes or one sliced jalapeno pepper. For a curried flavor, add ½ cup of coconut milk and 2 tablespoons of curry powder in between adding the remaining ingredients and the celery.

Turnip Hash Browns

Potatoes are often a staple in breakfast meals as hash browns or home fries. They are also high in carbs and starch. Turnips or rutabaga can be a good alternative: not only are they low in carbs, but they are also high in fiber and nutrients and flavor. They can be shredded similarly to potatoes to make hash browns in a skillet or baked in the oven. Spices, herbs, and salt can enhance the taste. Eggs are usually used to bind the shredded vegetable together, along with flour, though these ingredients can be easily switched to a lower-carb option:

- 1 medium rutabaga or turnip
- 2 tablespoons of water
- 1 tablespoon almond flour
- Dash of salt
- Black pepper

With a large shredder, grate the turnip or rutabaga into large shredded pieces. A smaller, finer grater can be used, though a large one will create a better texture for frying on the skillet. In a medium bowl, combine the grated turnip with water, flour, salt, and pepper and mix thoroughly until it is moist and slightly sticky. On medium-low heat, warm a skillet and pour some olive oil. Scoop two tablespoons of the mix onto the hasted skillet. Flatten gently with the back of the spoon and fry for 2 minutes.

Using a spatula, carefully flip the patty over and continue to fry for another 2 or 3 minutes.

What if the patty falls apart? Not a problem! Simply chop up the turnip mix and continue to try evenly, turning the mixture over until golden and slightly crispy. Serve as a side with smoked tofu and tofu scramble or on its own with a generous dollop of coconut yogurt.

There are other options to enhance the flavor:

- Add 1-2 tablespoons of very fine diced onion or garlic
- Fresh or dried herbs: dill, rosemary or paprika
- Spice it up with chili or cayenne pepper

Mix the desired option(s) into the batter before frying. Dried herbs can also be sprinkled on top as a garnish.

Protein Peanut Butter and Chocolate Breakfast Bites

These are quick and easy on-the-go breakfast bites that can be made within a few minutes or the night before. It's best to prepare at least two hours in advance to ensure they can chill in the refrigerator. This recipe includes peanut butter, which can be substituted for hazelnut or almond butter (they both have similar consistencies and work just as well). The ingredients are simple and easy to find in bulk or the dried goods area of the grocery store:

- 1 teaspoon MCT or coconut oil
- 2 cups of peanut butter
- ½ cup coconut flour
- ¼ cup low-carb sweetener (monk fruit or stevia)
- 1 cup melted dark chocolate (unsweetened) or cocoa

Prepare a medium or large baking tray (or similar-sized tray) by placing a baking or parchment paper. Place MCT or coconut oil, peanut butter, coconut flour, and sweetener in a medium bowl and combine. Mix thoroughly until all of the ingredients are evenly combined. Form small ball shapes and refrigerate for approximately one hour or freeze for 15 minutes. While the energy balls chill, prepare the chocolate by melting the equivalent of 1 cup dark, unsweetened (keto-friendly) chocolate or cocoa on low heat. Add a teaspoon of coconut oil and mix with a fork as the chocolate melts. If you have a powdered cocoa powder instead, this can be prepared by mixing with melted coconut oil (one or two teaspoons) in a small bowl. Add more chocolate or cocoa until there is enough to coat each one of the balls. When they are ready, remove them from the refrigerator or freezer and evenly coat each of them with chocolate and set aside. Once they are all coated, chill for at least half an hour, and they will be ready to enjoy.

If you want to get creative with these bites, they can be sprinkled with crushed peanuts, almonds, pistachios, or coconut flakes. Adding a dash of sea salt is another great option, for a "salted" taste.

Tofu and Spinach Breakfast Pies

These are prepared using an oven and a muffin tray with cup liners. Just like the egg and spinach bites or small pies, this recipe substitutes with tofu and spinach. These can be made the night before, refrigerated, and easily reheated in the morning. If made in the morning, give yourself some extra time to prepare and gauge how much time you need, especially if you have a busy schedule.

Just as with tofu scramble, this recipe works best when the tofu is marinated the night before. Although this is optional, it will create a stronger taste and provides a good way to infuse different spices with the tofu to soak overnight, as well as in the preparation the next morning. The ingredients are as follows:

- 1 block of tofu
- 1 teaspoon black pepper
- ¼ cup of vegetable broth
- ½ cup frozen (thawed) or fresh spinach (chopped)
- 2 tablespoons turmeric (add more to marinate with vegetable broth the night before, as well as when preparing the pies)
- 1 teaspoon diced onion
- 1 teaspoon sea salt
- Optional spices: thyme, dill, paprika, chili pepper

The oven must be ready at 350 degrees before baking. Prepare a muffin tray by placing cup liners (either disposable or reusable). In a medium bowl, add the block of tofu and mash with a fork. If marinated the night before, drain and keep ¼ cup of the fluid (broth with your choice of spices) or simply add the same amount of broth at that time and mix together. Continue to mash the tofu until it resembles a scrambled-like texture. Add the spinach, black pepper, salt, turmeric, and onion. It desired, add another 1 or 2 tablespoons of broth. Mix together thoroughly and transfer into a blender. Mix until as smooth as possible, then scoop to fill each muffin liner halfway. The recipe should yield approximately six pies. Bake for approximately 12-14 minutes, or until the texture resembles a mini quiche. If needed, bake for another 5-6 minutes. Garnish the top with dill or parsley and serve warm, or chill it and serve within the next 2 days.

Fruit and Keto Granola With Coconut Milk

This is an easy dish to prepare by simply combining the ingredients and enjoying with cold coconut (or almond) milk in the morning. The granola recipe under "snacks" can be added to this dish, or the following items can be dry roasted, cooled, and added to the milk.

- ¼ cup almond slivers
- ½ cup coconut flakes (unsweetened)

Roast the almonds and coconut in a skillet on medium for approximately 2-3 minutes until the ingredients brown, then remove it from the stove and add in a tablespoon of chia seeds and any other seeds or nuts you desire. Or you can simply add 1 cup of the vegan keto granola recipe to 1 cup of fresh fruit, and pour some coconut milk to cover most of the mix to enjoy. Dark chocolate or cocoa chips can be added as a topping.

Crispy Flaxseed Waffles

If you have a waffle iron, it doesn't have to be ignored once you switch to a vegan keto diet. This recipe is a new way to put this appliance to work, while providing a nourishing meal:

- 1 teaspoon baking powder
- 2 cups ground flaxseeds
- ½ cup water (separate)
- ½ cup avocado oil, olive oil, or coconut oil
- 1 teaspoon sea salt
- ¼ cup warm water combined with 3 tablespoons ground flaxseeds
- 1 teaspoon cinnamon or cardamom spice

Combine and mix the flaxseeds, baking powder, salt, and cinnamon or cardamom spice thoroughly in a medium bowl. Blend the wet ingredients (water, oil, and flaxseed-water mixture) in a food processor or blender until frothy, then add to the bowl of dry ingredients (already mixed). As these two batches of mixed ingredients are stirred together, they will thicken (this is exactly what you want to happen!). Heat the waffle iron and pour the batter to coat the inside, then close the lid and cook. Once the waffle is done, serve with coconut cream, low-carb syrup, or cinnamon powder. Fresh berries are another excellent option.

Vegan Keto Porridge

If you crave the comfort of a warm bowl of porridge or hot cereal, especially on a cold morning, this grain-free, low-carb recipe will provide that fix. As with many keto recipes, hemp hearts and flaxseeds are used to replace oats and other high-carb grains. Non-dairy milk is also added:

- ½ cup hemp hearts
- 1 cup of almond or coconut milk
- 2 tablespoons chia seeds
- 1 tablespoon monk fruit
- ¼ teaspoon vanilla extract
- ¼ teaspoon of cinnamon
- Dash of salt
- 3 tablespoons ground flaxseeds

Combine all the ingredients, including the non-dairy milk and refrigerate overnight in a sealed container. On the next morning, pour the ingredients into a small or medium cooking pot and heat on low to medium heat, stirring all of the ingredients until the cereal is brought to boil. Once it is ready, remove from heat and serve topped with slivered almonds or coconut flakes.

Pumpkin Pancakes

These are simple and easy to prepare for a unique spin on regular breakfast or weekend brunch. This recipe requires low-carb flour and canned or fresh pumpkin puree:

- ½ cup of pumpkin puree (canned or fresh)
- 1 teaspoon cinnamon
- 1 teaspoon nutmeg
- 1 teaspoon monk fruit (optional)
- 1 cup coconut milk
- 1 cup almond flour
- ½ cup coconut flour
- 2 tablespoons coconut or olive oil

Pour some olive or coconut oil in a warmed medium-sized skillet, and keep it on medium heat while you prepare a large bowl where you combine and mix all the ingredients. Use an electric or handheld whisk for best results. Blend well and avoid leaving any lumps or clusters of dried ingredients. Add a few teaspoons of water if the batter seems too runny for you. If it's too thick like a paste, add one or two tablespoons of almond flour. The batter should be thin enough to pour onto the skillet to make a 3-4-inch diameter pancake. Fry the batter for 1-2 minutes on each side. Serve with a sprinkle of cinnamon, nutmeg, fresh fruit, low-carb syrup, and coconut cream.

Cocoa Crepes Cocoa Crepes

If you enjoy dessert for breakfast, this is one option to consider. These crepes simply add cocoa powder to a simple three-ingredient vegan keto recipe as follows:

- 1 cup coconut milk
- ¼ cup cocoa powder
- 1 cup almond flour
- 2 tablespoons coconut or olive oil
- 1 cup coconut flour

Warm the skillet on medium-high heat, and pour the oil of your choice. While heating the pan, prepare all ingredients, and place them into a large bowl. Using a wire whisk or handheld mixer, and mix thoroughly all the ingredients to create a batter that is thinner or more runny than the pancake. Pour the batter into the skillet and cook for 1-2 minutes on each side. Serve with coconut cream or sprinkle with cocoa.

Pumpkin Protein Breakfast Smoothie

Bananas are often added to smoothies for their thickening effect. Pumpkin puree can provide a low-carb replacement for bananas in recipes. In this smoothie, pumpkin and almond butter provide a strong boost of fiber and protein to start off the day:

- 1 cup coconut or almond milk
- 2 tablespoons almond butter
- ½ cup pumpkin puree
- 2 tablespoons low-carb sweetener

Combine all ingredients in a blender and mix well for 30 seconds to one minute. Serve for breakfast or before a workout.

Almond and Pistachio Power Bars

These are energy bars that are made raw the night before and chilled for best results. The ingredients are simply blended in a food processor.

- 1 cup almond butter
- 2 teaspoons low-carb sweetener (monk fruit or stevia)
- ½ cup ground pistachios
- 2 tablespoons almond flour
- Dash of sea salt
- ½ teaspoon MCT oil

Prepare all ingredients and then combine and mix in a large or medium bowl. Make sure all the ground nuts and dry items are blended well into the almond butter using a fork. Prepare a small, square baking pan by adding the mixture and evening spreading to all sides and corners. Refrigerate for at least two hours, then remove and slice into bars. These are best made at night and refrigerated until the morning.

Other variations on this recipe include added shredded coconut or substituting pistachios for crushed walnuts or pecans. Almond butter can easily be switched to peanut, hazelnut, or sesame butter.

Tofu Berry Smoothie

Many recipes involving tofu require the firm or extra firm variety. Soft tofu is also an option for soups, sauces, and puddings. It can usually be found alongside many other tofu and meat-free options in the produce aisle. If you plan to use soft tofu, avoid choosing flavored puddings or desserts, as they are high in sugar. This smoothie adds a plain, unsweetened soft tofu to blend with berries. Since tofu is already high in protein and calcium, there is no need to add any supplements:

- 1 cup tofu
- 1 cup berries (fresh or frozen, any variety or mix)
- 1 teaspoon low-carb sweetener
- ½ cup almond milk

Combine ingredients in a blender and mix well for 30 seconds to one minute before serving.

Snacks

When going on a diet, including vegan ketogenic, it doesn't have to mean skipping snacks. Snacking in between meals or when you need an extra jolt of energy can be a great way to add more nutrients to your daily intake. There are plenty of tasty options, as well.

Kale chips

Baked kale chips are a delicious and healthy snack that's very easy to prepare. Kale is naturally bitter to taste, but that is nothing compared to its goodness. It contains plenty of vitamins, in addition to iron and calcium. One bunch of kale (any variety: black, green, or purple) can be used for chips. Any texture, from flat to extra curly is acceptable, as long as each piece is evenly coated in olive oil. The recipe only requires three main ingredients:

- One bunch of kale (any variety)
- Salt (sea salt or pink Himalayan salt is preferred)
- Olive oil (avocado or coconut oil is also acceptable)

Remove the stems from a bunch of kale and slice the leaves into small, 1 to 2- inch bite-sized pieces. If you need to wash the kale, make sure it is thoroughly dried before proceeding to the next step. While preparing the kale leaves, warm the oven to 350 degrees. Coat each piece of kale evenly and lightly in olive oil.

Prepare a baking tray and line with parchment paper. Evenly space the coated kale pieces, then sprinkle salt over all of them. Bake for 10 minutes when the oven is ready. Depending on the oven and size of kale, the cooking time can vary from 8-11 minutes. Monitor the chips carefully, as they can burn easily, within an extra minute or so. A couple of small batches may be a good idea as a "trial run" to determine the exact timing for each batch. Once this is established, making kale chips is one of the easiest recipes, and the results are addictive!

There are variations on this recipe, while keeping them both vegan and ketogenic:

- Add cumin and garam masala as a dried spice, along with salt, prior to baking.
- Chili pepper is a great way to spice up these chips, either in place of salt or mixed with it.
- Vegan parmesan or other dried cheese can be used to coat the kale to create a more "cheese" chip-like flavor. This may take a minute or two longer to bake.
- Garlic powder or salt, onion powder, paprika, and other similar spices can be used in combination or on their own to customize the flavor.

The best thing about kale chips? They don't take long to bake and do not require a dehydrator, though this can be used if desired. Kale chips take a fraction of time from preparation to finish than other vegetables, such as zucchini and other vegetables. This is because of the low content of water or moisture in kale.

Guacamole

This avocado-based dip can be used as a side for breakfast, as a dip with homemade vegetable chips or simply enjoyed on its own. It's completely plant-based and versatile for any meal of the day. The best avocadoes to use are very ripe and soft so that the fleshy part of the fruit can be mashed and mixed well with the other ingredients. There are only a few items needed to make a tasty guacamole:

- 2 medium or large sized avocadoes
- 2 tablespoons of olive oil (MCT or coconut oil can be used instead, or one tablespoon of each)
- Black pepper and salt
- 2 tablespoons lemon juice (or lime, if you prefer)
- Cilantro or parsley

Slice both avocadoes and remove their pits and scoop out the fleshy inside to a small bowl. Mash the avocado flesh well so that it is as smooth as possible, then add the oil, lime, or lemon juice, pepper, and salt, and continue to mix it thoroughly so that all ingredients are combined evenly. Cilantro and parsley can be chopped finely and added to the mix and topped as a garnish.

Vegan Keto Granola

Granola is typically made with oats, which are very high in carbohydrates. There is a low-carb option, which includes mixing a combination of nuts, seeds, and dried coconut flakes. There are some variations to this mix, which can be enjoyed as a cold cereal, with milk or coconut cultured yogurt, or as a topping on a dessert. The ingredients are easy to find, and can usually be found in bulk stores and regular supermarkets:

- 1 cup pumpkin seeds (toasted or plain)
- 1 teaspoon baking powder
- Dash of salt
- ½ cup hemp hearts
- ½ flaxseeds (whole or crushed)
- ¼ cup chia seeds (any variety)
- 1-2 tablespoons cinnamon
- 1-2 tablespoons psyllium husk and collagen powder
- ½ cup sunflower seeds
- Dried coconut flakes or shredded coconut (unsweetened)
- 1 cup of water

Before preparing the ingredients, start the oven and heat to 325 degrees. Prepare a baking sheet by lining it with parchment or baking paper. Place and grind all the seeds using a food processor or similar equipment. When the seeds are in smaller pieces (not powdered), mix in the remaining dry ingredients (everything but the water). Mix all of the ingredients evenly, then add the water and coat everything. Let sit for a few minutes to allow the granola to absorb the moisture. Spread the granola mixture evenly and thinly over the parchment paper and bake for 45 minutes. Monitor around 40-45 minutes, then remove from heat and break apart the granola with a spoon or spatula and bake for another half an hour (30 minutes). The mixture should be fully dry and crispy and ready to use once it is cooled. Remove from the oven and break up further, then store in a resealable container or use once it has cooled.

Keto granola is a tasty as a snack or a quick breakfast. It can be transferred to a reusable container as a snack on the run or enjoyed at home. This snack provides a lot of fiber and protein, which is ideal for a vigorous workout. For a more transferable snack option, other ingredients can be added to make it more of a "trail mix":

- Peanuts (raw or roasted)
- Almonds (slivered or crushed along with the cereal ingredients)
- Cocoa powder (sprinkled over the granola mix before baking – or used in place of cinnamon)

- Dried berries (unsweetened). Berries are typically low in carbs and can be added fresh or sun-dried in small amounts for a flavor boost
- Cardamom powder (instead of cinnamon)
- Sesame seeds

Chocolate Sesame Breakfast Smoothie

If you need a powerful boost in the morning, this is a simple and nutritious way to get it! Sesame butter is used in this smoothie instead of more common nut butters, such as peanut or almond butter. Sesame butter, or tahini, is commonly used in hummus and contains a lot of protein. Dark, unsweetened chocolate or raw cocoa can be used along with almond or coconut milk (or a combination of both):

- 2 cups almond or coconut milk (or one cup of each)
- 2 tablespoons of tahini or sesame butter
- ¼ cup dark chocolate unsweetened or raw cocoa (powder or melted in one teaspoon of coconut oil on low heat)
- 2 teaspoons monk fruit, stevia, or low-carb sweetener
- 2 teaspoons MCT or coconut oil
- 2-3 ice cubes

Place all the ingredients in a blender, placing the ice cubes last. Blend it for half a minute or so, until it runs smooth according to your favored consistency. Test the taste to decide if more sweetener is desired. This smoothie is also a good source of energy before a workout.

Coconut Bacon

If you crave bacon and miss the crispy flavor it provides, this recipe is an excellent alternative to substitute the real thing. This recipe involves smoking the coconut to create the distinctive flavor:

- 2 tablespoons of liquid smoke
- 1 tablespoon of soy sauce (unsweetened, no additives)
- 1 tablespoon liquid maple flavor
- 1 tablespoon water
- 3 cups of coconut flakes (unsweetened)

Before anything else, set the oven to 350 degrees temperature. In a medium bowl, combine liquid smoke, soy sauce, maple flavor, and water and mix. Add the coconut flakes and coat them evenly in the sauce, using a spoon to turn all the flakes to make sure they are all covered. Place a parchment paper on a medium or large baking sheet; spread the coated coconut flakes evenly on the sheet. Bake for 25 minutes and flip the flakes once every 5-7 minutes to ensure they all cook evenly. Remove from the oven once cooked, and allow it to cool before enjoying as a snack. They can be stored in a vaccum container or similar for up to 3-4 weeks or in the refrigerator.

Coconut Berry Smoothie

This is an easy way to get a boost of flavor and energy. This is prepared using coconut milk, fresh or frozen berries, and a low-carb sweetener:

- 2 cups unsweetened coconut milk
- 1 cup fresh or frozen berries (any variety or combination of strawberries, raspberries, blackberries, and blueberries)
- 1 tablespoon or sesame butter (for added protein)
- 2 tablespoons low-carb sweetener (stevia or monk fruit)

Blend all the ingredients for approximately 30 seconds to one minute. Remove once thoroughly blended to test the taste. Add more sweetener or other ingredients as desired. This smoothie is a great snack that can go into a portable cup for a road trip or commute to work.

Roasted Pumpkin Seeds

If you are planning on watching a movie or needs a light snack, this is a perfect way to replace chips or other high-carb options. During the autumn season when pumpkin is readily available, use the leftover seeds instead of discarding them:

- 2 cups of raw, dried pumpkin seeds
- 2 tablespoons olive oil
- Himalayan sea salt (enough to coat the seeds)

To get started, set the oven's temperature to 350 degrees and warm it up while you prepare the ingredients. In a large bowl, add the pumpkin seeds and olive oil, mixing well to ensure all seeds are coated. Add more oil if needed. Spread all the seeds on the baking sheet lined with baking paper and add some salt as desired. Place in the oven to bake for 10-12 minutes (more or less, until they are brown but not burnt). Roasted pumpkin seeds can be served after they have cooled a few minutes or stored and enjoyed up to 1 month.

Cinnamon Pumpkin Seeds

These are a variation on the regular roasted seeds, with sweetener and cinnamon instead of salt:

- 2 cups of raw, dried pumpkin seeds
- 2 tablespoons olive or coconut oil
- Cinnamon and low-carb sweetener (monk fruit is best) – just enough to coat the seeds

Follow the same recipe instructions for the regular roasted pumpkin seeds, coating first with low-carb sweetener, followed by cinnamon, or mixing both the cinnamon and sweetener in a bowl and coating the seeds with the blend. Bake at the same temperature and time frame until ready.

Rosemary Crisps

These are better than regular potato chips and with more flavor. Rosemary offers a unique taste to these crackers that pair well with vegan cheese, avocado, sliced tomatoes, and other toppings.

- 1 ½ cups almond flour
- ½ cup coconut flour
- ½ cup chopped pecan nuts
- 2 teaspoons baking soda
- 1 tablespoon fresh or dried rosemary
- ¼ cup ground flaxseeds
- 1 ¾ cups coconut milk (unsweetened)
- 3-4 tablespoons low-carb sweetener
- ¼ cup sesame seeds
- 1 teaspoon salt

Warm up the oven to 350 degrees. In a large or medium bowl, place both flours, salt, and baking soda and mix until well-incorporated. Add the sweetener and coconut milk and continue to stir. Then, add the remaining ingredients and continue to blend. Prepare one large baking sheet or two sheets by coating them in olive oil. Pour the batter the size a potato chip on the sheet and place in the oven. cook for approximately 30 minutes or until the crisp is in a golden brown hue. Remove from the oven and cool before serving. It is much easier to bake them thinner. If not consumed right away, it can be kept in an airtight bag in a pantry. They can be toasted or reheated in the oven if desired.

Lunches

Vegan keto lunches can be an easy meal to prepare for work, school, or at home. If you plan on eating at a cafeteria or nearby restaurant, keep in mind your options for keto and low-carb meals that are compatible with both a low-carb and plant-based diet. More restaurants and eateries, more than ever, are embracing new and modified menu items in response to a growing demand for both vegan and ketogenic meals and diets. The following food options can be found on many lunch menus:

- Vegetarian burgers, either soy or vegetable-based. If possible, note the brand and ingredients, as some plant-based burgers contain high-carb ingredients.
- Salads are a good option. Avoid sugary dressings and opt for balsamic vinegar or lime or lemon mixed with olive oil instead. Add nuts and seeds, and skip the cheese and dried fruit. Fresh berries are good.
- Side dishes may offer simple, healthy, low-carb, and vegetable options that can be combined (two or three) to make a complete meal. Examples of these are stewed spinach, pan-seared asparagus, fried zucchini, and baked squash. If you skip the main meal section of the menu and skim the sides, you'll be pleasantly surprised by some of the options available.

Preparing lunch in advance will not only help your budget; it will also keep you on track with the right food choices. There are many opportunities for lunch that are easy and light yet filling and satisfying.

Avocado and Tomato Salad

This is an easy and nutritious salad to prepare. The key to keeping the avocado from turning brown is by adding lime and olive oil. This can be prepared the night before, though it will be fresher if prepared earlier in the morning on the same day it is enjoyed. Choose the ingredients as fresh as possible. If the avocadoes are not ripe, they can still be sliced and added to the salad. These ingredients are easy to find and are best when they are in season or locally harvested whenever possible.

- 1 ½ cups of cherry tomatoes, sliced in half (as fresh as possible)
- 1 bunch arugula diced into small pieces
- 2 large avocadoes (if they are more firm than ripe, they can still be used, depending on your preference)
- 4-5 basil leaves, sliced (preferably fresh, or dried)
- 1-2 red, orange or yellow peppers sliced lengthwise

Combine and evenly mix the ingredients into a medium or large mixing bowl. In a small bowl, prepare the dressing by mixing the following ingredients:

- 1 tablespoon olive oil
- ½ teaspoon pink Himalayan salt
- 2 tablespoons balsamic vinegar
- 1-2 tablespoons lime or lemon juice

- ½ teaspoon black pepper
- 1 teaspoon of low-carb sweetener (preferably monk fruit)

Mix all of the ingredients and test the taste to ensure it is flavored to your desired level of sweetness or flavor combination. To serve the salad immediately, pour dressing over the salad and enjoy. If taking to lunch or consuming later in the day, add some lime or lemon juice to the salad to preserve the avocado, package the dressing in a small container separately, and mix just before eating.

There are some options to change the up the flavors to this dish. One option is to add roasted eggplant as a topping. To prepare the salad, slice a small eggplant into small disk shapes and rinse, then coat the slices in pink Himalayan salt, and set it aside for 20 minutes. Heat a skillet on low to medium heat. Rinse the eggplant slices in a colander once they have soaked in the salt for at least 20 minutes, which softens and prepares them for cooking. Fry on medium heat for approximately 5-6 minutes each side or until brown, then remove and add to the top of the salad. Zucchini can be similarly prepared in this way as an alternative topping, without coating in salt; simply slice the vegetable and fry it until golden.

Curried Tempeh and Snow Peas

Tempeh is fermented soy with a lot of nutrients and strong texture, making it a great feature of many dishes. In this recipe, the tempeh is marinated in curry spices overnight or for at least two hours before preparation. Snow peas can be either fresh or frozen. Other vegetables that work well in this dish include green peppers, asparagus, and zucchini, though these are optional (any low-carb vegetables can be added as desired):

- 2 cups of coconut milk
- 1/8 cup of curry powder
- 1 cup snow peas
- 1 tablespoon chili powder
- 1 block of tempeh (plain, unflavored)
- 1 tablespoon garlic salt
- ½ teaspoon black pepper
- 1-2 tablespoons of coconut or olive oil

Remove one block of tempeh from the package and slice into cubes. Combine the coconut milk, curry powder, and spices and mix well in a small bowl. Add the tempeh cubes to the bowl and make sure they are covered and coated evenly. Move all mixed ingredients to an airtight container and refrigerate overnight or at least for two hours to ensure they marinate the tempeh thoroughly.

When the tempeh is ready, heat on medium heat a pan or skillet with the oil of your choice. Drain the tempeh and retain the coconut milk and spice. Blend all of these in a small bowl. Fry the tempeh in the skillet, adding half of the coconut curry blend. Cook for approximately 10-12 minutes or until the tempeh is golden and slightly crispy. Add more of the coconut curry (or the remainder), and fry it for 2 minutes more before adding the snow peas. Fry the snow peas a bit; they still have to be crunchy when you serve them. Serve with salad or as a light meal on its own.

To enhance the flavor, garnish with crushed peanuts or sesame seeds. Fresh, chopped chives can also be added.

Avocado Toast

This can be an excellent breakfast, lunch, or brunch idea during a relaxing weekend. It involves using a keto bread of your choice (recipes in chapter 2) with vegan butter and fresh, ripe (not overripe) avocado.

- 2 slices of vegan keto bread
- 1 fresh, slightly ripe avocado, with both pit and skin removed and flesh cut into slices
- Vegan butter or olive oil (1 tablespoon)

Toast two slices of bread, and measure one tablespoon of olive oil in a small bowl or cup. Alternatively, vegan butter can be used instead of oil in the same amount. Coat both pieces of toast with butter (or oil), then cover in slices of avocado. Sprinkle with salt and pepper, then serve open-faced. If you want to add more to the overall flavor of the sandwich, top with fresh or dried basil leaves or sliced tomatoes.

Zucchini Noodles With Avocado Sauce

This dish combines spiral zucchini noodles or "zoodles" with a creamy avocado sauce, similar to Alfredo sauce. No cooking is required, and preparation is easy and fast, making this an ideal dish for lunch at work or over the weekend.

- 1 medium zucchini (spiraled into noodles)
- 1 cup dried basil
- ½ cup water
- 2 tablespoons of lemon juice
- 1 avocado (ripe)
- 8-10 sliced cherry tomatoes

In a blender or food processor, add the avocado, dried basil, water, and lemon juice and mix until smooth. Pour over the zucchini noodles on a plate and add in sliced cherry tomatoes. Sprinkle with basil and add dill if desired.

Fried Mushrooms and Brussel Sprouts

This dish combines a healthy portion of Brussel sprouts with mushrooms for a quick and easy skillet dish. If these vegetables are not your favorite, they can be substituted with asparagus or green beans for similar results. This meal is best served immediately after it is cooked:

- 1 cup of small mushrooms
- 2 tablespoons olive oil
- 1 teaspoon maple flavor
- 1 teaspoon sea salt
- 2 cups Brussel sprouts
- 1 tablespoon paprika
- 1 tablespoon vegan butter or coconut oil

Start the skillet on medium heat with some olive oil. Once warm and ready, cook the mushrooms for about 5 minutes, adding in the maple flavor, paprika, and sea salt. Continue cooking for another 5-10 minutes until the mushrooms are completely cooked and evenly coated in spices. Remove from heat and prepare a second skillet with vegan butter or coconut oil and preheat. Add the Brussel sprouts and water and cook until they are tender. That would be about 6-7 minutes. Drain, add the fried mushrooms, and combine. Serve warm.

Eggplant With Vegan "Cheese"

This is a simple version of eggplant parmesan, using vegan cheese as the substitute. To prepare the eggplant, slice into disk-like shapes, rinse in a colander, and coat evenly (both sides) with sea salt. Set aside for 20 minutes; the salt will soften the eggplant and prepare for the recipe. After 20 minutes, rinse in cold water and add to the recipe the following:

- 1 large eggplant, sliced into circles or disks
- Salt
- ½ almond flour
- ½ cup grated vegan cheese
- ¼ cup olive oil

Remove the prepared eggplant slices from the colander and coat lightly in olive oil. Mix and combine the almond flour and grated vegan cheese to coat the eggplant slices in a small bowl. Heat a skillet on medium and fry each slice on each side for about 5 minutes but not more than that. Byt then, they would be browned and ready to serve. Alternatively, the eggplant can be cooked in the oven at 350 degrees for 20-25 minutes or longer, depending on the size and thickness of the slices. Serve with soup, salad, or on its own as a light lunch.

Mediterranean Sandwich

This recipe works best with a light-textured vegan keto bread that can be easily toasted. For the Mediterranean flavor, a combination of olive paste, oil, and vegan cheese are used:

- Two slices of vegan keto bread
- 2-3 tablespoons of vegan cream cheese
- 1-2 tablespoons olive paste or pate
- 1-2 teaspoons olive oil
- Fresh basil leaves (as many as desired)
- ½ cup sliced cherry tomatoes

Toast both slices of bread and prepare the ingredients by mixing the olive paste and vegan cream cheese in a small bowl together. The olive oil can also be added to the bowl or simply used as "butter" for both slice of bread, whichever method is preferred. Spread the olive and vegan cheese blend on each slice of bread and top with fresh basil leaves and sliced cherry tomatoes

Tandoori Tempeh

This is a twist on the classic tandoori chicken dish, by simply replacing the meat with tempeh. For best results, marinate the tempeh overnight as follows:

- Slice tempeh into cubes, and add them to a bowl and coat in 2-3 tablespoons of tandoori paste

The following ingredients are used to make this dish:

- 1 ½ cups of coconut yogurt
- 3 tablespoons tandoori paste, unsweetened
- 1 teaspoon sea salt
- 1 block of tempeh (marinated and sliced into cubes)

Mix the yogurt and tandoori paste with the salt in a small glass bowl. Mix evenly and coat the tempeh cubes. Heat a skillet on medium and fry the tempeh until browned. Serve with salad or "riced" (grated) cauliflower or zucchini noodles.

Avocado and Tofu Bake

If you don't have time for breakfast, this is an option to prepare for lunch or late brunch. This recipe is simple. Scoop out the inside of an avocado, and stuff with the following ingredients:

- 2 tablespoons tofu scramble (recipe under breakfast) mixed with avocado
- 2 teaspoons dried or fresh dill or parsley
- Sliced green onions or chives for garnish

Combine ingredients inside the avocado shell and bake for 8-10 minutes. Serve with vegan keto toast or on its own.

Peanut Butter and Toast

This is a simple way to make your lunch if time is not available in the morning. The best bread to use is one with a thick texture and with lots of nuts and seeds. Peanut butter is a good source of protein, and it can be substituted with almond or hazelnut butter. Sprinkle cocoa powder as a topping.

Curried Broccoli and Kale Soup

This is a delicious lunch during a cold day that can be prepared the night before and reheated the next day. It is baked in the oven where all flavors combine and incorporate evenly. This meal combines two highly nutritious greens like broccoli and kale, with a curry flavor.

- 1 teaspoon garlic powder, plus 2 teaspoons
- 3 ½ cups grated or "riced" broccoli
- 3 tablespoons curry powder
- ½ teaspoon paprika
- 3 tablespoons olive oil
- 2 cups chopped kale; stems removed
- 1 teaspoon cumin powder or seeds
- 1 cup coconut milk
- 4 cups vegetable broth
- ¼ teaspoon sea salt
- 1 teaspoon black pepper
- Dash of salt or to taste

Combine and mix the broccoli, curry powder, olive oil, garlic powder, cumin, paprika, and salt in a medium mixing bowl. Spread the coated broccoli on a baking tray lined with baking paper, and roast them in the oven for 20 minutes. Remove, then set aside and prepare the soup. Chop the vegetables and measure the ingredients. Add the roasted broccoli mixture to the blender and mix. Prepare a large cooking pot where you add onion, oil, and 2 teaspoons garlic powder and sauté for 4-5 minutes. Add the vegetable broth and milk, vegetables, and broccoli "rice," along with the spices. Allow it to boil and then lower the heat, cooking on medium for 20 minutes. Garnish with parsley and bread and serve warm.

Sesame Tofu Bake

This is an easy, almost snack-like lunch that can be prepared in advance and made available for a quick, light meal.

- 2 teaspoons sesame oil
- ½ block extra firm tofu
- 1 cup vegetable broth
- 2 teaspoons sesame seeds

Slice the tofu into cubes. Pour the vegetable broth in a small or medium glass bowl and add sesame oil. Add the tofu to a resealable container and pour the broth and oil mixture over the cubes and marinate in the refrigerator overnight or for at least two hours. When ready to bake, warm the oven at 350 before preparing the other ingredients. Prepare a small baking pan with the drained tofu. Retain some of the liquid to pour over the tofu cubes, and sprinkle them with sesame seeds. Bake for 20 minutes until browned and serve.

Curried Cabbage

This is a fast and simple dish that requires little preparation, with the exception of slicing half of a head of cabbage, which can be done with a knife or shredder.

- 2 tablespoons tomato paste
- 2 tablespoons curry powder
- Half of a cabbage, sliced into thin leaves, stems removed
- 2-3 tablespoons olive oil

On medium-high heat, pour some oil in a skillet and add curry powder. Fry for one minute, then add the tomato paste. If the paste does not spread into the curry and oil, add an extra tablespoon. Add the cabbage slices and fry on medium heat until all of the cabbage has softened and is coated with the oil, curry, and tomato paste mix. Smoked tofu, fried onions, and mushrooms can be added to this dish.

Pizza Stuffed Peppers

If you have an extra green pepper or two, this recipe is a good way to make use of the pepper's shell, by stuffing and baking it as a "pizza."

- 2 green peppers, cut in half, seeds removed
- 2 cups vegan cheese
- 1 cup tomato sauce
- Optional spices: oregano, paprika, dill, parsley
- Sea salt and pepper
- Meat-free pepperoni (optional)
- Spinach

Fill each pepper with the following ingredients, in this order: a thin layer of tomato sauce, followed by vegan cheese, spinach, and meat-free pepperoni (one or two slices per green pepper "half"). Add salt and pepper on top and sprinkle with extra vegan cheese. Bake for 5-10 minutes in the oven. These can also be heated in the microwave.

Grilled "Cheese"

This recipe requires no major preparation, once you have your favorite vegan keto bread and vegan cheese chosen.

- One or two slices of vegan cheese
- Avocado, sliced (optional)
- 2-3 tablespoons olive oil
- Two slices of vegan keto bread

Warm a skillet with olive oil on medium heat. Add a thin layer of oil on one side of each bread slice, and add cheese, avocado, and other ingredients before forming the sandwich and frying on both sides until crispy and brown. Serve with a few slices of tomato or dill pickles or both.

Smoked Tofu and Arugula Salad

Smoked tofu can be found in the produce, meat-free area of your supermarket. It can also be prepared similarly to the sesame-baked tofu dish, only with liquid smoke in place of sesame oil. For convenience, smoked tofu can be purchased and is often available in several brands. Always choose the option with the least additives:

- ½ block of smoked tofu
- 1 lime squeezed
- 2 teaspoons olive oil
- Arugula, chopped

Pour some lime juice over the arugula in a mixing bowl and some olive oil and mix evenly. Toss and add a dash of sea salt (optional). Layer the smoked tofu over the arugula and serve.

Lettuce Wrap Sandwich

This is a sandwich or wrap option that eliminates bread altogether. To prepare a lettuce wrap, simply slice off large leaves of lettuce and form a taco-shaped wrap to fill with any of these ingredients:

- Vegan cheese slices
- Smoked tofu or another meat-free slice
- Pesto (dill, parsley or rosemary)
- Roasted eggplant
- Fried mushrooms
- Grilled portobello mushrooms

There are many more options to consider. Wrapping your lunch in lettuce is a way to add more fiber into your meals.

Tofu "Bacon," Fried Onions, and Avocado Sandwich

If you search in a few natural food stores, supermarkets, and, sometimes, local markets, you may find a soy-based bacon alternative. Smoked tofu is another option. This sandwich is full of flavor and can be reheated or toasted just before adding the ingredients. Fried onions can be caramelized by adding a low-carb sweetener, such as monk fruit in place of sugar. The avocado slices are added first, followed by the tofu bacon, then topped it with fried onions.

Fried Zucchini with "Cheese"

This recipe is as easy as slicing one or two zucchinis lengthwise and adding them to a heated skillet with olive oil. Fry on both sides for approximately 1-2 minutes on medium heat until slightly golden, then remove and serve with shredded vegan cheese.

Cream "Cheese" Bagel

The vegan keto breakfast bagel can work wonders in lunch options. A simple toasted bagel with vegan cream cheese is an easy way to enjoy lunch.

Vegan Deli Bagel

This bagel sandwich combines several sliced vegan "meat" and "cheese" flavors, along with other toppings, such as tomatoes, olive paste, avocado, and pickles. Hot peppers, salt, and black pepper are great options.

Spinach Guacamole Bagel

The guacamole recipe under "Snacks" is a great addition to any sandwich. Mixing the guacamole with raw or cooked spinach in between a bagel would provide more iron and minerals.

Smoked Tempeh, Mustard, and Arugula Bagel

Combining the sharp flavor of mustard, smoked tempeh (or tofu), and arugula is another option for using the breakfast bagel.

Spinach, Walnut, and Avocado Salad

If a light lunch suits your schedule best, this quickly put-together salad can keep you fed while you work or allow you to enjoy more of your lunch.

- 1 cup raw, washed spinach
- 1 tablespoon olive oil
- ½ cups crushed walnuts
- 1 ripe avocado
- 1 tablespoon lemon juice (or lime if you prefer)

In a small mixing bowl, place the lime or lemon juice with the olive oil, and set to the side to mix well. Place all the other ingredients in a large or medium bowl, then add the salad dressing and toss. Serve with soup, if available, or as a quick meal on its own.

Roasted Almonds and Walnuts on Arugula

Pan-roasted almonds and walnuts, with little or no olive oil, can be tossed with arugula for a simple, light salad. Combine 1 teaspoon balsamic vinegar, dried rosemary, and 1 teaspoon olive oil to create a dressing to add.

Stuffed Peppers and Wraps

These can be oven-baked, or if you're in a hurry, they can be heated in the microwave. Add baked tofu slices, curried tempeh, and any variety of finely chopped vegetables to use as stuffing for the peppers. They can also be an ideal wrap or taco for many other ingredients and recipe creations.

Dinners

Whether you need to replenish after a busy day, or you want to impress guests with a delicious dinner, there are plenty of options that fall under the vegan keto diet. These recipes will make a positive impact on anyone, even if they do not follow a plant-based and ketogenic diet.

Vegan Keto Moussaka

This dish is traditionally prepared with meat, which can be simply replaced or omitted in this recipe. Moussaka is a rich meal and also tasty comfort food. This is a simplified version of the recipe to adapt to the vegan keto diet:

- 1 cauliflower (ground or mashed into small pieces; riced cauliflower will work)
- 5 cloves of garlic (crushed)
- 1 eggplant slices into cubes
- Vegan cheese, shredded
- Sea salt (just a dash to taste)
- Vegan moussaka sauce (combine in a bowl and set aside):
  - 1 can tomato
  - 1 block of tempeh
  - 1 tablespoon onion powder
  - ¼ cup tomato paste
  - 1 tablespoon wine vinegar

o   Dash of salt and pepper

Grate the cauliflower (or use "riced" cauliflower) and cook until tender in a medium-sized pot with ¼ water. Drain and mash the cauliflower heads, add garlic, and set to the side. While preparing the cauliflower, the oven must be warmed to 350 degrees. Prepare the remaining ingredients. Line a baking dish with olive oil and begin to layer with the following: cauliflower mash as the first or bottom layer, followed by the next layer of vegan moussaka sauce. Continue to add layers of tempeh, eggplant slices, vegan cheese, and so on, ending with the top layer, which should be mashed cauliflower sprinkled with vegan cheese. Bake for 25-30 minutes and serve warm.

Zucchini "Zoodle" Pasta and Tomato Sauce

This is a twist on the simple spaghetti and tomato sauce dish, which is often served with meatballs as the main meal. It can also be served on the side if you want variety. In this recipe, the spaghetti noodles are replaced with zucchini noodles or "zoodles," which are prepared by spiral-slicing a raw zucchini into long spirals. Vegetable noodles are becoming popular and more readily available in grocery stores in the produce aisle. This meal is simple, with noodles and a tomato sauce, which can be the base for other toppings and ingredients.

- 3-4 cups spiral zucchini noodles, or two medium-sized zucchinis
- 2 tablespoons garlic powder
- 1 tablespoon oregano
- 2 cups of tomato sauce (unsweetened; if you use canned tomato sauce, check to confirm there are no added sugars or carbohydrates)
- 1 teaspoon chili powder
- 2 teaspoons tomato paste
- ½ teaspoon sea salt
- 2 tablespoons dried basil

Prepare the zucchini noodles with a spiral slicer or use zoodles that were prepared ahead and add to a large colander. Rinse and set aside. Heat a medium cooking pot with tomato sauce and paste and stir in the spices, keeping the heat to low-medium for 10 minutes. This recipe will serve 3-4 portions. Add zucchini noodles to a small or medium plate and pour tomato sauce. Add shredded vegan cheese as a topping.

Vegan "meat" balls or soy-based ground "meat" can be added to the tomato sauce as it stews. When choosing a meat alternative, review the ingredients to rule out additives and sugars, which may be present in some brands. Pan-seared tempeh, prepared in a skillet, can be a great way to add protein to this pasta dish.

Broccoli and Cauliflower Fried Rice

"Riced" cauliflower is popular due to its mild flavor and consistency, which can replace rice in most dishes. Broccoli can also be a good replacement instead of cauliflower or combined together. To "rice" these vegetables, divide the head of cauliflower and broccoli into quarters or smaller for them to fit a food processor. You can also use a blender to grind and blend and them until they resemble a fine, rice-like texture and size. A grater can also be used in place of a food processor. The following ingredients, similar to regular fried rice, are also included:

- 1 teaspoon of garlic powder or finely ground fresh garlic
- Dash of pink Himalayan salt
- 1 small shallot or onion, finely and thinly chopped or grated
- 1 tablespoon olive, avocado, or coconut oil
- Dash of black pepper
- ¼ teaspoon of grated ginger root
- 1 teaspoon of sesame oil
- 4-5 tablespoons of chopped parsley or cilantro
- Slivered almonds

Warm a skillet on medium heat (or low heat) and add some oil of your choice. Add the riced cauliflower and broccoli, along with the garlic, to the pan and cook for 1-2 minutes, mixing occasionally. Add some salt and sesame oil and continue to fry for another 2 minutes, then add the grated ginger root. Cook for another 2 minutes or until the riced vegetables are mostly cooked but not mushy and still a bit crunchy. Serve and garnish with cilantro or parsley and slivered almonds.

This is a basic fried "rice" dish that can be served as a main meal with one of the following toppings:

- Fried mushrooms. Any variety, including shitake and portobello. Grilled portobello or regular mushrooms would make an excellent topping.
- Fried red onions
- Roasted almonds on the skillet. This can be prepared in advance and later added to the rice dish as a topping.
- Grilled eggplant

Portobello mushroom burgers

The strong, "meat-like" texture of portobello mushrooms make them an excellent substitute for meat or other vegetarian burger options. These burgers can be served with a vegan keto bun (or bread) on top of lettuce or on their own with toppings. During a summer barbeque, these are best grilled with other vegetables, including zucchini and eggplant. These burgers can be prepared on a barbeque grill or skillet:

- 2 portobello mushrooms
- ¼ cup balsamic vinegar
- 1 teaspoon dried basil
- Dash of salt and pepper
- 2 tablespoons olive oil
- 1 teaspoon dried oregano

Prepare the barbeque to grill portobello mushrooms by brushing with olive oil and preheat. Put the oil, pepper, balsamic vinegar, oregano, salt, and basil in a small mixing bowl and mix and set to the side. Grill for 5-6 minutes on each side, brushing the mushrooms with the marinade on both sides when switching.

If preparing in a skillet, heat on medium with olive oil and fry the mushrooms for 6-7 minutes on both sides, coating each side with the balsamic marinade. When the burgers are done, serve on a keto bun or a bed of fresh spinach sprinkled with fresh lime and balsamic dressing.

There are many topping options for portobello mushroom burgers:

- Skillet fried or raw sliced onions
- Sliced green pepper (fried or raw)
- Vegan cheese
- Smoked tofu (sliced and topped on the burgers)
- Lettuce (as a bun or topping)

Vegan Keto Lasagne

Lasagne can be easily switched from the high-carb original to a vegan keto version with a couple of simple changes: switching the noodles for cabbage and omit the meat (or add a vegan alternative). This is a meal that can vary considerably according to your favorite vegetables and flavors.

- 2 tablespoons olive oil
- One head of cabbage (medium)
- 2 zucchinis sliced thin, lengthwise
- 1 cup of spinach
- 2 cups of tomato sauce (plain, no additives)
- Vegan cream cheese
- 2 tablespoons shredded vegan cheese (cheddar or mozzarella)

Before any preparations, warm up the oven to 350 degrees. Wash the vegetables with running water and cut them up. Evenly coat with some olive oil a large baking pan and spread a thin layer of tomato sauce. Add cabbage leave slices over the tomato sauce layer, and make sure all of the stems are removed before doing so. Ensure the cabbage covers the pan evenly, and add another layer of vegan cream cheese, then spinach, tomato sauce, another layer of cabbage, then more cheese, tomato sauce, zucchini, and continue to layer until either cabbage or zucchini is the top layer.

Sprinkle lightly with olive oil and cover in shredded vegan cheese. Bake for 40 minutes and serve warm.

Other ingredients to add include vegan ground "meat," which can be added as a layer. Vegan shredded cheese is another option.

The Ultimate Vegan Keto Platter

This is an ideal dinner idea for an event or when you expect guests. All of the following ingredients are arranged on a large, oval-sized serving platter:

- Dill pickles, sliced lengthwise
- Fried mushrooms
- Smoked or pan-seared tofu (in cubes or slices)
- Cauliflower and broccoli (cut into small florets)
- Vegan cheese slices
- Black olives
- Grilled zucchini (or fried for 5-6 minutes on a skillet)
- Fresh berries
- Dried coconut pieces
- Celery sticks

Cauliflower "Macaroni and Cheese"

The original macaroni and cheese dish can be adjusted to the vegan keto version by substituting the macaroni for cauliflower and adding vegan cheese. For this recipe, add more than one type or flavor of vegan cheese to increase the variety and strength of taste for this dish.

- 1 head of cauliflower
- 1 teaspoon of paprika
- 2 cups shredded vegan cheese (cheddar flavor)
- ½ cup almond flour
- ½ cup vegan dried or "parmesan" cheese
- ¼ cup olive oil
- 1 cup shredded vegan cheese (mozzarella flavor)

Warm up the oven on 350-degree temperature while you prepare everything else. Slice the head of cauliflower into small pieces, approximately ½ to 1-inch in size. Using some olive oil, grease a medium-sized rectangular baking pan and add half of the cauliflower. Combine the cheddar and mozzarella-flavored vegan cheeses and blend in a medium mixing bowl, then add a layer of half of the cauliflower over the bottom layer. Add the remaining cauliflower to the cheese mix and combine and add to the rest of the pan. In a second small bowl, mix the dried vegan cheese and almond flour. Coat the top of the casserole with the dry mix. Sprinkle with paprika. Bake for not more than half an hour. By then, the top should be golden, but it would be better to check every 10 minutes. Serve warm.

Vegan Keto Chili

Skipping the meat, cheese, and beans in a pot of chili may seem like a change to a completely different dish altogether, though there are some great options for preparing a healthy chili that is both low in carbs and free of animal products. Chilis are best cooked slowly. When you have time to stew, add and stir ingredients for two hours. In a large cooking pot, add 4-6 cans of diced tomatoes on low to medium heat, along with any spices you wish to add (salt, pepper, chili pepper or flakes, oregano, paprika, etc.). The following ingredients may be considered:

- Chopped celery
- Spinach
- Chopped onions
- Crush garlic
- Diced green peppers
- Vegan ground "beef"
- Okra, chopped
- Jalapeno peppers
- Mushrooms
- Zucchini

Once the chili is ready to be served, garnish with vegan cheese.

Vegan Keto Bruschetta Bread

This recipe is best prepared with a natural-tasting vegan keto bread. It is very similar to regular bruschetta using the following ingredients:

- 6-8 slices of bread
- 2-3 tablespoons olive oil
- 3 tomatoes
- 1 small onion, finely chopped
- ½ cup of freshly chopped basil leaves
- 2 teaspoons balsamic vinegar
- 1 clove of crushed garlic.
- Salt and pepper.

Before preparing the ingredients, heat the oven to 350 degrees and then line with parchment paper a baking tray. Add the bread to the tray and coat them lightly in olive oil. Warm the bread until toasted (about 10 minutes) and transfer on another tray to cool. Combine and mix well the rest of the ingredients in a bowl. Coat each slice of bread with these toppings and serve. This bruschetta recipe goes well with chili and soups.

Roasted Butternut Squash

This is a simple recipe that can fulfill a meal with a tasty, mouth-watering vegetable. It's a dish that's best enjoyed at home, as it is prepared in the oven and enjoyed as soon as it's ready:

- 1 medium butternut squash (if not available, another squash variety will work)
- Salt
- Olive oil

Warm the oven to 350 degrees before preparing the squash. Line a baking sheet with paper suitable for baking. Rinse butternut squash with cool water and slice in half. Lightly coat both halves in oil and sprinkle with salt. Bake for approximately half an hour and enjoy.

<u>Butternut Squash Soup</u>

If you are in the mood for soup, use the recipe for roasted squash using the following:.

- 3 tablespoons olive oil
- Roasted butternut squash, peeled and chopped into smaller pieces
- Dash of salt
- 1 celery stalk, thinly sliced
- 1 teaspoon black pepper
- Thyme
- 1 small onion, grated or thinly sliced
- 3-4 cups vegetable broth

Place all the ingredients into a medium cooking pot on medium-high heat. Wait for it to boil before removing from the heat to cool. Transfer the contents to a food processor, blending in batches, if needed, until smooth. Return soup to the pot and reheat until ready to serve. Garnish with thyme.

Curried Pumpkin Soup

This soup is created similarly to butternut squash, replacing the squash with pumpkin puree and adding curry powder and coconut milk.

- 3 tablespoons olive oil
- 2 cups pumpkin puree
- 1 teaspoon black pepper
- 1 celery stalk, thinly sliced
- 2-3 tablespoons curry powder
- ½ cup coconut milk
- 1 small onion, grated or thinly sliced
- Dash of salt
- 3-4 cups vegetable broth

Combine all ingredients into a large cooking pot and allow to boil under a medium-high flame. Just after boiling, remove from heat. Transfer to a food processor when cool and blend. You might need to do it in batches until the soup is smooth or according to desired consistency. Return the soup to the pot and reheat until ready to serve.

Cream of Asparagus Soup

This is a delicious soup that pairs well with salad, bread, or a baked vegetable. It can be a side dish or a main meal.

- 2 tablespoons olive oil
- 2 lbs of asparagus, chopped into small, bite-sized pieces
- Sea salt
- Black pepper
- 3-4 cups vegetable broth
- 1 clove of garlic, minced
- ½ cup almond or coconut milk
- Chives and dill for garnish

Prepare and warm a large saucepan or pot. Add the olive oil under medium flame and add garlic. Cook for 1-2 minutes and then add the asparagus, pepper, and salt. Continue to cook and add the broth when the asparagus is tender. Simmer the broth for another 10 minutes, then remove from the heat to cool. Move to the blender and process in batches until all is done. Return to the pot to reheat. Serve with dill or chives as a garnish.

Cream of Cauliflower Soup

The same delicious and creamy soup can be adapted for cauliflower.

- 2 tablespoons olive oil
- 1 head of cauliflower, chopped into small, bite-sized pieces
- Sea salt
- Black pepper
- 3-4 cups vegetable broth
- 1 diced onion
- ½ cup almond or coconut milk
- Paprika

Set a large cooking pot over a medium flame on the stove. When warmed, add some olive oil, followed by the garlic, and cook it for 1-2 minutes. Add the cauliflower, pepper, salt and continue to cook until the cauliflower is soft. Add the broth and simmer for about ten more minutes. When cooked to your preference, remove from the heat to cool. Move to the blender and process in batches, when needed, and return to the pot to reheat. Serve and garnish with paprika.

Skillet Meals for Dinner: The Easy Way to Vegan Keto

There are many options for stir fry dishes that can fit into any lifestyle or way of eating, including a plant-based ketogenic diet.

The following recipes are various skillet meal combinations that can be served on their own, with zucchini noodles, or "riced" broccoli or cauliflower. All skillet meals are prepared using olive oil:

Skillet Meal 1: Tofu, Spinach and Garlic

This is a simple but effective way to get a lot of nutrients and good boost to your immune system without many ingredients. Once the skillet is heated, add the tofu first, followed by garlic then spinach. Mushrooms can be added at the end if desired.

Skillet Meal 2: Tempeh, Cabbage, and Onions

Tempeh is a powerful source of nutrients, including B12. Cabbage and onions make a good fit, as they are both strong in flavor and enhance the dish.

Skillet Meal 3: Cauliflower, Garlic, Ginger, and Green Beans

Before you begin, crush the garlic and ginger and sauté lightly, then add the green beans and cauliflower.

Skillet Meal 4: Asparagus, Garlic, and Mushrooms

Any variety of mushroom will work well with this dish. Always add mushrooms last, as they cook faster than the other vegetables. Add sesame seeds for extra flavor.

Skillet Meal 5: Bell Peppers, Okra, and Eggplant

Add extra salt to soften the eggplant, and add okra last, as it cooks faster than the other ingredients.

Skillet Meal 6: Artichoke, Spinach, and Mushrooms

Artichoke and spinach work well in dips and sauces, and their flavors also complement one another in this skillet. Mushrooms are another good way to enhance the overall taste of this dish.

Skillet Meal 7: Brussel Sprouts, Vegan Butter, and Garlic

These powerfully nutritious vegetables can stand on their own with some garlic and butter or combined with other vegetables. They are delicious as an oven-roasted dish sprinkled with vegan cheese and sea salt.

Skillet Meal 8: Asparagus, Almonds, and Garlic

Garlic is consistently a good option for skillet meals and a good way to boost your immune health. Almonds can be slightly toasted and slivered before adding to this meal. Top with vegan cheese.

Skillet Meal 9: Celery, Green Beans, and Almonds

This is simply pan-seared green beans added to celery and roasted almonds.

Skillet Meal 10: Baked Sesame Tofu, Snow Peas, and Garlic

This prepared tofu can be sliced and fried with garlic and snow peas.

Skillet Meal 11: Bok Choy, Broccoli, and Garlic

This combination works best with some soy sauce added, though this is optional. Garlic and olive oil will bring out the flavors in these vegetables as well.

All skillet meal ideas are guides only and can be simply combined or changed according to individual taste and preference.

Desserts

Chocolate Avocado Mousse

This dessert requires only three ingredients and can be made within 1-2 minutes. If you have a craving to satisfy, or you simply want to create a simple and easy dessert on short notice, this is the perfect option.

- One very ripe, large avocado
- 2 tablespoons dark, unsweetened cocoa or dark chocolate powder (melted dark chocolate also works in this recipe)

Combine the avocado and cocoa in a small mixing bowl. Mash the avocado, incorporating the cocoa powder until smooth and blended. Serve immediately in a small dessert bowl (makes 1-2 servings). Add a topping, such as whipped coconut cream that is sweetened with stevia or monk fruit.

Cinnamon and Almond Cookies

This is a good option for comfort food, especially when you are craving something sugary or high in carbs. These cookies are baked in the oven and only require five ingredients:

- 2 cups of almond flour
- ¼ cup low-carb sweetener (stevia or monk fruit)
- 2 tablespoons of chia seeds
- 2 tablespoons cinnamon powder
- 3-4 tablespoons freshly squeezed orange

To start, warm up the oven to 350 degrees. Grind the chia seeds to smaller pieces using a food processor. Add the sweetener to incorporate well with the chia seeds. Add to a medium bowl with the remaining ingredients and mix everything together. A thick dough will form, which should provide enough for 7-8 small cookies. Roll into small half-inch balls and put on a paper-lined baking sheet. You can create other shapes, or you can simply make balls that you can flatten with a spoon or fork. Bake for 14-15 minutes.

Fat Bombs: A New Way to Treat Yourself on the Vegan Keto Diet

Fat bombs are healthy fat fuel treats that can be prepared quickly and with only a few ingredients. They are usually stored in the freezer or refrigerator and reserved for when you need that sweet fix or treat. Once you try a few fat bomb recipes, you'll want to experiment with more ingredients, flavors, and ideas for new combinations. Before you begin, you'll need a few items to get started:

- Small-sized muffin tray
- Reusable liners (single-use paper liners can be used, though reusable is recommended)
- Ice cube tray

Chocolate Peanut Butter Cups Fat Bombs

If you love chocolate and peanut butter together, this is a win-win recipe. It only requires three ingredients:

- 1 cup of peanut butter (unsweetened)
- 1 cup melted dark, unsweetened chocolate or cocoa
- 2-3 tablespoons monk fruit or stevia

When melting the chocolate, add the monk fruit or stevia and stir in thoroughly. Half of the melted chocolate will be used for the bottom layer and the remainder for the top, with the peanut butter in the center. Prepare a muffin tray (small size is ideal, any size will work), and add one layer of melted chocolate to the bottom of each liner, up to one third, then store for 20 minutes in a chiller or freezer. When ready, add the second layer (peanut butter) for another third of each cup, then return to the freezer. After another 20 minutes, add the final layer of chocolate, and freeze it again for another 20 minutes. The cups are now ready to enjoy. They should either remain in the freezer or can be kept in the refrigerator until eaten, as they will melt quickly at room temperature.

Coconut Fat Bombs

These treats are one of the best ways to increase healthy fat in your vegan keto diet. All of the ingredients are coconut-based. MCT oil can be added with the coconut oil (an extra teaspoon) to increase the fat amount further.

- ¼ cup coconut butter
- ¼ cup coconut oil (or 1/8 coconut oil and 1/8 MCT oil)
- 2 tablespoons shredded coconut, unsweetened
- 1 teaspoon monk fruit or stevia

Combine all the items on the list in a glass bowl, and mix everything until the sweetener is completely dissolved and incorporated with the other ingredients. Scoop the blend into an ice cube tray or small silicone molds and freeze or refrigerate for 10-15 minutes.

Strawberry "Cheesecake" Fat Bombs

These are tasty bite-sized strawberry cheesecake fat bombs made with vegan cream cheese and fresh or frozen strawberries:

- ¼ cup coconut butter (peanut or almond butter)
- ¼ cup vegan cream cheese
- 2-3 tablespoons coconut oil
- 3 tablespoons low-carb sweetener
- ½ cup sliced strawberries

Combine the ingredients in a small bowl and mix well. Scoop into silicone moulds or a muffin tray and freeze for approximately 20 minutes, then enjoy.

Pistachio Fat Bombs

- 2/3 tablespoons coconut oil
- ¼ cup pistachios (ground)
- 1-2 tablespoons low-carb sweetener

Combine and mix ingredients in a small bowl, making sure all of the ground pistachios are blended into the coconut oil and sweetener evenly. Scoop into silicone molds or a muffin tray and freeze for 15-20 minutes.

Almond Fat Bombs

- 2-3 tablespoons coconut oil
- ¼ cup almond butter
- 1-2 tablespoons ground almonds
- 1-2 tablespoons low-carb sweetener

Mix all of the ingredients in a glass bowl and transfer to a muffin tray or silicone molds. Ground almonds can be omitted or substituted with slivered almonds or almond meal if desired. Freeze for 20 minutes before consuming.

Chocolate Fat Bombs

If you simply love chocolate, these are a delicious option for a quick snack.

- ¼ cup coconut butter
- ¼ cup cocoa powder or melted dark, unsweetened chocolate
- 2 teaspoons coconut oil
- 1-2 tablespoons low-carb sweetener

Combine ingredients and mix well. If you are using melted chocolate instead of cocoa powder, heat a small pan on low heat and melt chocolate until it is even without any lumps before mixing. Both cocoa powder and melted chocolate can be used together in this recipe, for a double-chocolate effect. Shredded coconut is another option if you enjoy coconut and cocoa combined.

Pumpkin Fat Bombs

When pumpkins are in season, use this recipe as an easy way to use up any leftover fresh pumpkin, or you use the canned version.

- 1 teaspoon cinnamon
- 2 tablespoons pumpkin puree
- 2 teaspoons coconut oil
- 1-2 tablespoons low-carb sweetener
- 1 teaspoon nutmeg
- ¼ cup coconut butter

In a mixing bowl, medium in size, combine and mix well all ingredients on the list. Add an extra tablespoon of pumpkin puree, and increase cinnamon and nutmeg spices if desired. Pour mixture into silicone molds or a tray and freeze for at least20 minutes.

Cardamom-Cinnamon Fat Bombs

A unique and tasty option for fat bombs, the combination of both cinnamon and cardamom create a delicious treat. If you prefer one spice more than the other, simply remove one and double the preference:

- 2 tablespoons coconut oil
- ½ teaspoon cinnamon
- ½ teaspoon cardamom
- ½ teaspoon low-carb sweetener (optional)
- ½ teaspoon vanilla extract
- ¼ cup finely shredded coconut

Combine and thoroughly mix all the ingredients in a small bowl and place on a muffin tray or silicone molds to freeze for at least 15-20 minutes.

Vegan Keto Brownies

Brownies are a great dessert and snack at the same time. The ingredients in brownies can be changed to suit a variety of flavor and dietary options. The key to successful brownies is keeping them moist and soft:

- ½ coconut butter
- 6 tablespoons low-carb sweetener
- 2 teaspoons flaxseeds combined with 4 teaspoons warm water (in a small bowl)
- 1 teaspoon baking powder
- 1 teaspoon vanilla
- 1 cup almond flour
- ¾ cups cocoa powder
- ¼ cup ground walnuts or almonds

Preheat oven to 350 degrees. Combine all of the ingredients in a large bowl and blend thoroughly, making sure there are no lumps. Prepare a square or rectangular baking dish. Grease with olive oil and add the batter, spreading it evenly across the pan. Bake for 15 minutes.

Cheesecake Cup

This recipe is prepared raw, with no baking or cooking required. All that is needed is a tall glass and the following items layered from bottom to top:

- 2 tablespoons almond flour mixed with 1 teaspoon low-carb sweetener
- 1 cup vegan cream cheese, blended with monk fruit and 1 teaspoon of coconut milk
- Add fresh fruit, cinnamon, or cocoa powder on top of the cup
- 1 teaspoon vanilla extract (added to cream cheese and sweetener)

Pumpkin Cheesecake Cup

Apply the same recipe used for regular cheesecake cups. This recipe varies from the previous one when you combine ¼ cup of pumpkin puree with the vegan cream cheese. This cup can be garnished with nutmeg and cinnamon.

Cocoa Cheesecake Cup

Replace the ¼ pumpkin puree with the same portion of cocoa powder or melted dark, unsweetened chocolate. The topping can be cocoa powder, cinnamon, or a combination of both.

Lemon-Lime Cheesecake Cup

Add 1 tablespoon of lime juice and 1 of lemon juice into a small bowl and combine, then add to the regular cheesecake cup recipe.

Fruit Salad

Keto-friendly fruits tend to be few, though there is a good combination of low-carb fruits that can be enjoyed in small doses. These fruits can be added "as is" or chopped into smaller, easy-to-eat sizes for one serving:

- Kiwi
- Strawberries
- Lime and lemon juice (combined, 1 tablespoon)
- Firm and slightly ripe avocado slices

Dark Chocolate and Berries

Some dark, unsweetened or similar low-carb chocolate options are a great fit for the vegan keto diet. One bar of this specialty treat can be expensive, though only a small amount is needed to melt and pour over berries or other desserts like crepe or ice cream. Dark chocolate, when melted, can be an excellent dip for fruits.

Vegan Keto Ice Cream — Cocoa and Vanilla

This is a one-serving ice cream recipe that combines the following few ingredients.

- 1 tablespoon cocoa powder
- 2 tablespoons monk fruit
- 1 teaspoon vanilla extract
- 1 cup coconut milk

Combine and mix all the ice cream ingredients in a glass mixing bowl, and pour the contents to a jar or wide container and freeze.

Vegan Keto Ice Cream — Cinnamon

Combine all the ingredients from the above recipe, and substitute cocoa powder for cinnamon. Cardamom may be used in addition to cinnamon or as a replacement.

Drinks

Cardamom and Ginger Spice Tea Drink

This is a delicious, warm drink that can be enjoyed during cold weather or as a late-night treat before bed. The base can be water, green tea, or coconut milk

- 2 cups of coconut or almond milk (or water with green tea)
- 2 tablespoons dried ginger root
- 2 tablespoons crushed cardamom pods
- 2 tablespoons low-carb sweetener

Add and mix all the ingredients to a small cooking saucepan and bring to a boil on low heat, while stirring in the spices and sweetener. Once it is ready, serve it warm with a cinnamon stick.

Matcha Green Tea Latte

Matcha green tea is a delicious tea that is full of antioxidants. It can simply be prepared by steeping green tea powder or leaves in a cup of hot water to serve with or without sweetener.

A latte is prepared using milk, and in this drink, either almond or coconut milk can be used as a base. If you don't have a latte or espresso machine, this drink can be prepared on a stovetop by boiling the milk and adding the following:

- 2 tablespoons matcha green tea powder
- 2 cups coconut or almond milk
- 2 tablespoons low-carb sweetener

Bring all ingredients to a boil on low to medium heat and serve in a mug.

Regular Coffee With Almond Milk and Sweetener

If you are a coffee drinker and enjoy this way of getting your caffeine fix, simply brew your favorite blend of coffee and add almond milk and your favorite low-carb sweetener, similar to adding cream and sugar, only without the dairy and carbs! Coconut milk is another option, though almond milk tends to mix better with coffee.

Iced MCT Coffee

MCT oil or coconut oil can be added to a hot cup of coffee or any other beverage to increase the amount of healthy fats in your diet. Iced coffee is an easy way to get a dose of MCT oil while spicing up the drink with cinnamon, low-carb sweetener or cocoa powder. One or two teaspoons of MCT oil or coconut oil is all that's needed. Almond milk can also be added, along with ice, and blended for a tasty treat.

Cucumber and Lime Water

Water infused with natural flavor is a great way to quench your thirst during the warmer months or a vigorous workout at the gym. All that is needed is a large jug of filtered or spring water, one lime cut into quarters, and 5-6 slices of cucumber. Chill overnight or for several hours to flavor the water and serve with ice.

Lemon and Mint Water

Like the cucumber and lime water drink, this flavor option is the same, only with fresh mint leaves and lemon. Lime can be substituted for lemon if desired.

Vegan Keto Eggnog

A holiday favorite, eggnog is usually very high in sugar and dairy, though it is a drink many people look forward to during the festive season. In this recipe, the dairy is replaced with coconut milk, which is thick and tasty for this beverage. Maple or vanilla flavoring can be added, though this is optional:

- 2 cups coconut milk
- ¼ cups water
- 2 tablespoons vanilla or maple flavor
- ½ teaspoon nutmeg
- ½ teaspoon cinnamon
- ½ cup raw almonds or cashews

Soak the almonds or cashews overnight in ¼ cup of water so they become tender. If you want to create this drink in a shorter time frame, the minimum soaking time is one hour. When the almonds or cashews are ready, combine with the rest of the ingredients in a blender and mix for one minute. Serve chilled.

Berry juice

If you have a juicer, a blend of berries combined with water is a cool, refreshing treat in the summer. This recipe is easy to create with a handful of fresh berries (about 1 cup) and 1-2 cups of water. Add to a blender and mix until all of the berries are blended well. Add ice cubes and serve.

Chapter 8: Bonus Chapter: Enjoying the Vegan Keto Diet and Recipes Without Expensive Ingredients

How do you save money and budget on the vegan keto diet? Food is often expensive, and with so many options and places to choose from, sticking with a budget is difficult. Balancing the grocery budget only becomes more challenging with a new diet. As with any way of eating, there are ways to reduce and control spending to get the most out of your money while sticking with a healthy vegan keto diet:

- Prepare a list of basic goods that you need every week, and "build" or add more food items according to your expenses for food. Allow some extra funds for extra items or unexpected increase in some items.

- Buy in bulk. This is especially a good idea for snacks and baking ingredients. Avoid the higher costs of goods from packaging and buying more of one item than you want or need. Choose 2-3 recipes and note the measured amounts of each ingredient to use as a guide for the purchase. For example, if you only require a ½ cup of almond flour, buy 1-2 cups in bulk instead of purchasing a full package, unless you have a lot of baking planned. For large volume baking and cooking, buying in bulk may or may not be advantageous, depending on the types of items you need. Research ahead and compare prices whenever possible.

- Keep it simple. The most expensive foods are often processed or packaged and not the healthiest option. These types of foods are usually chosen for snacks. Even protein bars, low-carb pastries, and other goods claim to be ketogenic and vegan, but they are usually overpriced and may contain hidden sugars and other ingredients that can hinder your progress. There are plenty of easy recipes for homemade versions that can be prepared, many without baking or too many ingredients. You can also get these at a fraction of the cost.
- Choose whole foods. Ditch the packaged kale chips for fresh kale, and make your own snack. Scoop a handful of raw almonds instead of potato chips. Find a fresh, natural alternative for snacking to replace old habits. This may take time, although it will be healthier and cheaper overall.

Chapter 9: Vegan Keto Diet for Long-Term Success in Health and Weight Loss Goals

Succeeding at the vegan keto diet is all up to how well you can adapt and follow new food choices, learn about nutrients, and avoid processed and high-carb foods. Making notes, researching new products, learning about the different vegetables and fruits (both local and imported) are part of a new approach to diet. Such a diet does not focus on the restrictions but on the opportunities of trying many new foods. The information in this book provides a foundation and guide to start you on the right path to achieving a sustainable and long-term diet plan that will result in a better way of living and eating for life.

Conclusion

Thank you for making it to the end of *Vegan Keto Diet: The Ultimate Ketogenic Diet and Cookbook, With Low-Carb and Vegan Keto Bread Recipes to Maximize Weight Loss and Special Ideas to Build Your Keto Vegan Meal Plan.*

Let us hope it was informative and able to provide you all of the tools you need to achieve your goals, whatever they may be.

The next step is to work on your diet and take action!

Finally, if you found this book useful in any way, a review on Amazon is always appreciated!

KETO CHAFFLE RECIPES

The Ultimate Ketogenic Diet Cookbook with Low Carb and Snacks Recipes to Lose Weight and Boost Your Metabolism. Sweet and Delicious Ideas to Prepare Keto Desserts

By Tyler Allen

© Copyright 2020 Tyler Allen
All rights reserved.

This document is geared towards providing exact and reliable information with regards to the topic and issue covered. The publication is sold with the idea that the publisher is not required to render accounting, officially permitted, or otherwise, qualified services. If advice is necessary, legal or professional, a practiced individual in the profession should be ordered.

- From a Declaration of Principles which was accepted and approved equally by a Committee of the American Bar Association and a Committee of Publishers and Associations.

In no way is it legal to reproduce, duplicate, or transmit any part of this document in either electronic means or in printed format. Recording of this publication is strictly prohibited and any storage of this document is not allowed unless with written permission from the publisher. All rights reserved.

The information provided herein is stated to be truthful and consistent, in that any liability, in terms of inattention or otherwise, by any usage or abuse of any policies, processes, or directions contained within is the solitary and utter responsibility of the recipient reader. Under no circumstances will any legal responsibility or blame be held against the publisher for any reparation, damages, or monetary loss due to the information herein, either directly or indirectly.

Respective authors own all copyrights not held by the publisher.

The information herein is offered for informational purposes solely, and is universal as so. The presentation of the information is without contract or any type of guarantee assurance.
The trademarks that are used are without any consent, and the publication of the trademark is without permission or backing by the trademark owner. All trademarks and brands within this book are for clarifying purposes only and are the owned by the owners themselves, not affiliated with this document

200

Summary

INTRODUCTION 203

KETOGENIC DIET AND ITS HISTORY 205

WHAT IS KETOGENIC DIET? 211

BENEFITS OF KETO DIET 222

WHAT IS CHAFFLES? 243

HOW TO MAKE CHAFFLES 244

THE EFFECT WHEN KETO MEETS CHAFFLES 245

KETO DIET AND CANCER 256

KETO DIET AND EPILEPSY..................................271

KETO DIET AND BLOOD PRESSURE 273

WHAT DO I EAT ON A KETO DIET?.........................275

FOOD TO EAT ON A KETOGENIC DIET 276

FOODS TO AVOID ON A KETOGENIC DIET 279

BOOST YOUR METABOLISM 282

GETTING STARTED ON THE KETO DIET 295

TIPS AND GUIDELINES 300

KEY PILLARS GOING FORWARD..........................308

BREAKFAST AND BRUNCH CHAFFLES RECIPES....311

LUNCH AND DINNERS CHAFFLES RECIPES 347

BASIC FLAVORED CHAFFLES RECIPES 379

CONCLUSION 443

INTRODUCTION

Developed and introduced decades ago, the ketogenic diet has gained rapid recognition in recent years. The main reason the keto diet attracts appeal is primarily due to its novelty as it is distinct from a fad diet. While individuals who embrace the keto diet experience significant body developments, in addition to weight loss and body build-up, keto diets also provide numerous health benefits. Individuals are encouraged to consume foods with a keto diet that consists of the nutrients necessary for body growth while eliminating toxins that could harm the body system. The keto diet focuses on the consumption of low carbohydrates, which are essential for the body to recover quickly from body loss or weight loss after conversion to energy.

One may wonder how high a diet of carbohydrates is said to be harmful to personal health, and why should it be avoided? Carbohydrates are transformed into glucose when consumed, resulting in an increase in the insulin body. Insulin is released into the bloodstream to decompose the glucose that develops into the body system's main source of energy. An increase in the amount of insulin in the body system leads to an increase in fat storage. Therefore, lower carbohydrate quantities in a daily diet provide more fats to the body, which can be broken down to form body energy.

Another vital benefit derived from ketosis is the support that it provides the body with less food for survival. When in ketosis, due to the low availability of carbs in the body, the body becomes sensitive to the use of fats as the primary source of energy other than the use of carbs. The liver breaks down fats into ketones in ketosis, which helps the body use fats as energy. Ketosis also encourages adequate calorie consumption, while lower quantities of carbohydrates are required. It allows for weight loss to be faster and more normal. We would address certain essential health benefits that can be obtained from keto diet apart from weight / fat reduction later in the book.

The keto diet is not difficult, although misunderstandings exist about it. It can be challenging to start a keto diet just as it is difficult to start a new thing. One would, however, be overwhelmed by the intrinsic benefits of avoiding the consumption of carbs. Furthermore, it comes with great advantages to have portions of bacon on a diet.

KETOGENIC DIET AND ITS HISTORY

Fasting led some medical specialists to explore the idea of a ketogenic diet by mimicking the fasting concept, i.e. consuming zero calories. Even today, the people believe that fasting is the human body's best self-healing medicine. Fasting comes with a number of advantages and most are due to the presence of ketones in the body.

Fasting is believed to cleanse the body and soul, both physically and spiritually, and it is a practice that has been used by people for over a thousand years. Fasting in one form or the other is encouraged and endorsed by almost every religion and culture in the world. The ancient Greek philosopher, Hippocrates, mentioned fasting as the best medicine for healing oneself of sickness. He said—"Every disease begins in the intestine." Fasting will put your body into ketosis and people who performed fasting were not clearly aware of this crucial factor (ketosis). The state of ketosis in your body is the best natural anticonvulsant drug you can ever get. That was discovered by the Mayo Clinic doctors in the early 1900s. Fasting can bring down the seizure frequency in patients with epilepsy. But it is not practically possible to keep on fasting, especially with small children (affected by epilepsy). This is when the doctors noticed a linkage between fasting and low-carb diet. The doctors found that the number of epileptic seizures had diminished. A strict low-carb diet has nearly the same effect as convulsion fasting. When the scientists identified a way to measure blood ketone levels, a connection was established between the keto diet and the fast. By the mid-1900s they realized that fasting had led to the production of ketone in the body.

Medical practitioners soon started using the low-carb high-fat diet to treat epilepsy in both children and adults. The ketogenic diet has a variety of benefits, in addition to controlling seizures. The ketogenic diet helps regulate the insulin levels in the body and maintained this diet until 1921 when insulin was discovered; people suffering from diabetes. William Banting, a British mortician, advocated this diet as a weight loss diet after losing weight, in a book entitled Letter on Corpulence.

The fall of the Ketogenic Diet

This diet (low-carb high fat) was considered by many to be a counter-intuitive approach to health maintenance. Even today, many people are afraid that continuous high-fat food consumption can lead to high cholesterol levels, obesity, high blood pressure and various other health issues.

An American biochemist, Ancel Keys has published an epidemiological study which links dietary fat as the primary risk factor for heart disease. In this epidemiological study Ansel investigated how fat consumption increased heart disease development. The cholesterol and blood LDL derived from dietary fat speeds up the development of atherosclerotic plaque (the body stores cholesterol in blocking blood flow walls of arteries). His work was published at the time when he suffered a heart attack from the then US President Dwight Eisenhower.

After his doctor's advice, the President immediately cut his fat intake. This gave more power to the hypothesis of Ancel Keys and people started to view nutrition as a crucial factor. This has become the reason why the global food policy and its public practice have changed dramatically. Subsequently, the USDA (US Department of Agriculture) recommended a reduction in dietary fat intake for Americans in their dietary goals, and advised people to include a cereal-and grain-based diet.

But no clinical evidence was yet available to support Keys ' diet-heart theory during that period. A few large trials have been conducted to show that a decrease in dietary fat may decrease the risk of heart disease but they have all failed—including the Women's Health Initiative Randomized Controlled Dietary Modification Trial and the Framingham Study.

Following the new USDA recommendations for decreasing dietary fat, the rate of obesity grew as people began to follow the guidelines described. Few medical researchers pitched in and published hypothesis reports that showed that the recent development of health crisis is due to increased dietary carbs intake. The phenomena was identified by John Yudkin, the author of the book "Sweet, White and Deadly." The book spoke about the pervasive distrust of dietary fats that nutritionists and scientists have led them to almost ignore the role of starch and sugar in the body.

Comeback of the Low-carb diets

The idea of low-fat diet made its way around the late 1900s, after the diet-heart experiment was published by Ancel Keys. It was during this period that Dr. Robert Atkins came up with his low-carb diet version. In 1972, he published a book, Dr. Atkins ' Food Explosion, which spoke of a particular low-carb diet of similar shades of ketogenic diet. During his 40 years of practice he listed how he had treated around 60,000 patients (estimated count) for obesity and its associated conditions.

But no clinical studies or experiments were performed to affirm or verify the dietary benefits which he listed. Most of his patients reported various side effects beginning with the diet. The side effects of that were:

- Nausea
- Fatigue
- Dizziness
- Weakness
- Headache

Doctors classified these effects as Atkins Flu, because many people find the beginning step of the diet very unpleasant. A lot of people started promoting the keto diet for health after his death in 2003. It was during this period that a group of scientists (Dr. Eric Westman, Jeff Volek, and Stephen Phinney) supported the Atkins Foundation to systematically research the diet and its impact. They discovered that a diet based on the 1977 USDA guidelines that was outperformed by the Atkins diet. With respect to the measured coronary risk factors which included lower lipoprotein cholesterol and total blood saturated FFA, the high-density lipoprotein cholesterol was increased alongside.

What caused the result? It can be due to the reduced carbohydrate and its associated changes in hormone setup, or due to ketones on the metabolism of the body. With more people coming out to support the low-carb high-fat diet, the public perception began to change and the pendulum was swinging in its favor. Dr. Jason Fung, Professor Tim Noakes, and Professor Thomas Seyfried have published their work on keto diet, thus exposing the hypothesis defects in the diet-heart. Speakers and writers like Robert Lustig, Nina Tiecholtz and Gary Taubes have written for the low-carb diet.

The influencers revealed how political choices in favour of high-carb diets contributed to food attacks such as keto diets. More pieces of evidence pitched in to demonstrate the rise in diabetes rate and obesity due to high-carb diet. Also, multiple studies suggested continuous low-fat diets could be harmful to overall health. A recent meta-analysis of data from 18 countries associated with high-carb consumption with a rise in mortality rate achieved its climax level.

People who previously feared high-fat intake now started to fear high-carb intake and an increase in sugar levels. Following the ketogenic diet and its growth in popularity, the last few years saw a considerable increase in people. More people have begun adopting this new dietary pattern, and numbers of online searches corresponding to the ketogenic diet have grown.

Many people today follow the ketogenic diet to cure obesity and metabolic disorders. Thousands of people join big online forums to discuss the high-fat low-carb diet. By sharing their experiences before and after the diet they share their success stories thereby encouraging more people to adopt this dietary routine.

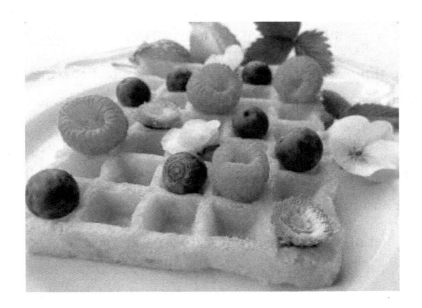

WHAT IS KETOGENIC DIET?

Learning what keto diet is enlightening. Keto diet can be described simply as a low-carbohydrate diet. Nonetheless, it is unique from other low-carb diets as it adjusts the meat, protein, and starch balance to ensure the fats become the body's main source of energy. Naturally, as its primary source of energy, the human body uses carbohydrates, leaving fats to accumulate in large quantities. The common way to reduce body fats is to combine proper body exercise with a reduction in the amount consumed, a means used to ensure that energy expenditure exceeds calorie intake. This is the biggest reason why many people on traditional diets never lose weight.

On the flip side, ketogenic diets turn fats into body fuel rather than fat accumulation, making it easier to lose weight. Ketogenic diets are also referred to as diets for regeneration, as it also eliminates illnesses such as diabetes, high blood pressure, obesity, heart disease, among others, due to the reduction of sugar consumption it promotes.

Manipulating fats, protein, and carbs to embrace ketosis is very important. This (ketosis) is a situation in which the body, other than dependence on sugar and carbohydrates, has to adapt to the use of fats as its main fuel. As a result, there is a substantial increase in protein and fats relative to the overall amount of carbs. Also, low carbohydrate consumption is accompanied by lower insulin quantities in the body, which translates into lower body fat storage and glucose. This explains why keto diets are the most preferred solution for diabetic patients as it regulates the sugar level in the body naturally.

The proportion of fats, carbs, and protein can vary as many consume about 50 grams of carbohydrates per day, resulting in weight loss at times. The quantity of carbs consumed can be approximately 15-20 grams per day under strict adherence. The weight loss can be accomplished over time by eating fewer amounts of carbs; nevertheless, the diet can be very supple.

The number of calories should not be counted during keto diet; the quantity of carbohydrates taken should be monitored while adjusting the consumption of carbs and fats & protein. A conventional keto diet derives its calories from 60, 15-25, and 25 percent of fats, protein, and carbohydrates. The downside of the plan, though, is the consumption of sugar that would be prevented. The ketogenic diet is different from that of a fad. The essential benefits and health solutions derived from ketosis have been demonstrated by various scientific studies. If you are interested in weight loss, less sugar intake, and proactive measures against susceptibility to critical health issues, you can talk to a medical practitioner.

What are Ketones?

Okay, what exactly do these ketones come from and where? As mentioned above, when your body exhausts its reserves of glucose (glycogen) it will be looking for another alternative source of energy. This is when it gets digging into the fat storehouse of the body as stored fat can help fuel your cells with the energy required.

Since there is no oxygen in the blood, the processed fats will be taken in by the liver and converted to fatty acids. These fatty acids then split into functional compounds known as ketone bodies (known as ketones). Your body uses those ketones to give your body cells and brain cells electricity. The best part is when blood ketone levels increase reducing the appetite. The explanation for increased energy is because the brain requires another source of energy to generate.

The liver contains three distinct types of ketone bodies:

- Acetoacetate
- Beta-Hydroxybutryate
- Acetone

The body can fuel itself from ketones in two different ways:

- Your body can make its own ketones by eating or by increasing the fat intake and reducing your carb intake by inducing carbohydrate abstinence
- You can also supply your body with real ketones by taking exogenous ketones (ketone supplements)

Once your body is on a ketogenic diet, it acts as a fat-burning engine. It inevitably leads to low insulin levels and the ability to consume fat rises as it becomes easy to access the fat stores. When it releases ketones, the body is in ketosis, and the quickest way to shift your body to ketosis is to fly. But for ever fasting is difficult, and this has led to the development of the ketogenic diet.

Is it possible to lose weight because the body enters into ketosis?

Once your body starts eating fat contained in ketones, your body changes to ketosis. But why is this going to bring me down weight? I understand from whence you come. Let me just give you an example of this.

Just pretend you've packed a load of coal for the winter ahead. When it's winter, some of these piles of coal are scooped up for heat into the furnace. The pile gets smaller as you start to use up all the fuel. Similarly, your body burns the stored fat in your body in ketosis and as it continues to make use of the stored fats (which is your extra flab, water weight, excess calories, etc.), you get smaller, i.e. you reduce weight. Here the coal is the stored fat and your energy is the heat you receive in winter.

There are numerous studies on how a well-planned ketogenic diet has helped many people lose weight by enhancing their fitness metrics and increasing their overall health status. Thermodynamics is another important reason to lose weight on the ketogenic diet! You get rid of one big macronutrient-carbohydrates-when you practice the keto diet!

The following list includes the carbohydrate rich food items:

- Soda
- Bagels
- Fruit smoothies
- Bread
- Sugar candies
- White rice
- Pasta

Such foods have a high caloric content, and those calories are stored as fat in your body when you over-eat. When these carb-rich foods are restricted or eliminated, you consume fewer calories. You loose weight when you burn more calories than you consume. This is one of the main reasons why most calorie-restricted diets cause weight loss when done correctly regardless of the amount of the food you eat. You don't concentrate on the body composition, food quality or muscle development on this type of diet but it's more about the amount of food eaten (smaller portions of food).

Once your body is accustomed to the keto regimen, you feel satiated with fewer calories, resulting in faster and easier weight loss in the process. Just note, you'll probably gain more weight if you overeat on a keto diet. Yeah, don't expect to lose weight daily after eating 6000 calories of ham, beef and butter! You need to know how to eat healthy!

The ketogenic diet assists in weight loss as well as helps in:

- Epilepsy treatment
- Type 2 diabetes
- Managing PCOS (Polycystic ovary syndrome)
- Treats acne
- Showing improvement in neurological diseases such as MS (multiple sclerosis and Parkinson's)
- Reducing the risk of cardiovascular and respiratory diseases

Researchers are doing more research to understand how the keto diet impacts Alzheimer's patients and similar health problems.

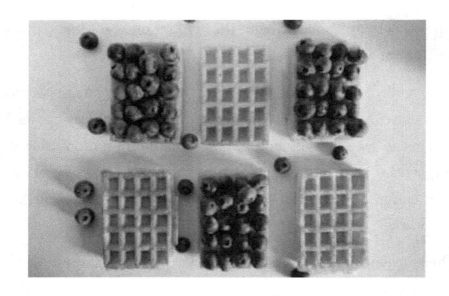

Types of Ketogenic Diets

There are various types of ketogenic diets and each comes with its own variations of the diet protocol. But the forms are familiar and popularly known:

- **Standard Ketogenic Diet (SKD)**

The Standard Ketogenic Diet (SKD) is what most people think when we talk about a keto diet. This is an extremely low carbohydrate diet, mild in protein and high in fat. If you are looking for quick fat loss and only do low to moderate intensity workouts (e.g., biking, running, yoga, and light weight lifting), then the SKD may be the best diet for you.

With this approach to diet, carbohydrates have to be greatly restricted. A daily intake of 30 g or less of carbohydrates is usually required in order to induce and stay in ketosis (which is one of the primary purposes for so much reducing carb consumption). Keto carb levels vary from person to person, but the general rule is to eliminate nuts, starches, added sugars and other high-carbon foods.

Low carb fruits, nuts, beans, and high fat dairy products will be the primary sources of carbs on the SKD.

- **Cyclical Ketogenic diet (CKD)**

The Cyclical Ketogenic Diet (CKD) is a nutritional method incorporating the day(s) of carb loading with the traditional ketogenic diet. It is usually used by those who are more experienced when it comes to exercise at high intensity. Bodybuilders and athletes are a perfect example of people who should use the CKD, as their preparation requires a high volume and strength to improve their output. With this tremendous volume and intensity, without the help of carbs, it is almost difficult for them to practice at their peak.

For this reason, it is best for them to implement carbohydrate refeeding days once or twice a week to fully replenish glycogen stores in order to fuel their training bouts with a sufficient amount of sugar.

Unlike the TKD, where the primary goal is to maintain a moderate level of blood sugar and muscle glycogen for training, the CKD's goal is to fully replenish glycogen during carb loads and deplete glycogen and increase ketone levels between carb loads. Both dietary strategies will however allow you to reap the benefits of carbohydrates and ketosis.

- **Targeted Ketogenic diet (TKD)**

The Targeted Ketogenic Diet (TKD) consists of eating carbs around workout times (usually 30-60 min before) and at any other time following the SKD. The TKD provides us with an easy way to maintain high-intensity exercise efficiency and facilitate glycogen replenishment over long periods of time without interrupting ketosis.

Usually, this dietary plan is prescribed for two specific groups of people: (1) individuals who need carbohydrates to sustain their exercise performance but are unable or unwilling to take part in a CKD's lengthy carb loads or (2) individuals who are just beginning an exercise program and are unable to do the amount of exercise required to maximize a CKD diet;

If you're doing just aerobic style workouts or any practice that's low to moderate in difficulty, then the TKD (and CKD) isn't for you— then stick to the SKD.

- **High-protein Ketogenic diet**

This diet resembles your standard ketogenic diet but the only difference is in the macronutrient composition ratio. The diet includes more protein, where the ratios are mostly 5% carbs, 35% protein and 60% fat.

Extensive studies on the standard and high protein ketogenic diets have been conducted. But the targeted ketogenic diet and cyclical ketogenic diet are advanced keto diet methods followed by bodybuilders or athletes.

When people refer to ketogenic diet they usually refer to the general standard ketogenic diet.

BENEFITS OF KETO DIET

While the ketogenic diet is widely recognized as a "rapid diet for fat loss," the crucial role that it plays in healthy living goes beyond weight loss. In reality, higher energy rates and weight loss are side-attractions compared with other huge benefits that can be obtained from the diet. Scientific studies have proven these advantages.

First of all, it should be noted that carbohydrate diets with their high quantity of sugar and other processed components do not offer any health benefits. These are common calories, and the majority of processed foods deny the body of nutrients needed for a healthy life. Below are the benefits for energy conversion derived from low carbohydrates and higher fat intake.

1. **Control of Blood Sugar**

Low body sugar levels are important to the treatment and prevention of diabetes. Keto diets have been known to be a very effective tool for diabetes prevention. Many patients with diabetes have enormous body weight, making weight loss a necessity. Meanwhile, in addition to what keto diet does, carbohydrates are converted into sugar, which is very harmful to patients with diabetes because it causes an increase in sugar levels. Therefore, low carbohydrate consumption virtually prevents such a spike in sugar and also regulates blood sugar levels.

2. **Mental Focus**

The keto diet is related to low carbohydrate regulation and increased fat and protein. As discussed, the body is forced to depend on fats as its main source of fuel generation. It differs from the traditional Western diet that is less nutritional, especially in fatty acids that are much required for good brain function.

When people experience deficiencies and cognitive disorders such as Alzheimer's, this implies insufficient glucose for brain use. The loss of insulin allows the energy level to decline, thereby increasing the brain's performance. The keto diet, however, prevents this deficiency as it provides additional energy to the brain.

The study also revealed that the keto diet could improve the memory capacity of people with Alzheimer's disease. The memory capacity of people affected by Alzheimer's is also proportional to the number of ketones in the body.

An average individual's interpretation of this information is that keto diet improves brain functionality, memory capacity, and overall brain health. This is due to the presence of fatty acids, namely fish omega 3 and omega 6. The brain tissue mainly consists of fatty acids (reason fish are referred to as "Brainfood"), which means that the use of such fatty acids will improve the brain's health. Our body does not produce fatty acids alone; only through our diet can we obtain them. And the diet of keto is full of fatty acids.

When on a diet with higher quantity of carbohydrates, the result can be a muddled brain, where it becomes less possible to focus on thoughts. However, increased energy in comparison to keto diets makes it easier to focus. In reality, for better brain performance, people who do not want weight loss follow keto diets.

3. **Increased Energy**

Poor carbohydrate-filled diets often result in weakness and fatigue following daily activities. Meanwhile, fatty acids are a better efficient source of energy, constantly renewing the body system, making one feel more energized and strengthened in comparison with the feelings of a "sugar" rush.

4. **Acne**

It appears surprising to many people when they get to know that keto diet also helps with healthy skin and elimination of skin acne. This is because it is not a pronounced benefit and not well-documented. While acne is a relatively common skin disease among adults, it is more prominent among teens as about ninety of them suffer from it. Acne, over time, has been perceived to be a result of poor diet; however, controlled research studies are ongoing to establish the authenticity of the claim. It has been proven that individuals on keto diet have clearer skin, which is free from acne. The logical explanation to this is that a 1972 study proved that large amount of insulin causes skin acne, which is being prevented by keto diets as it keeps insulin at a low and moderate level needed for healthy living, hence, improved skin health.

Also, inflammation causes acne. Meanwhile, keto diets reduce inflammation, which in turn helps the body in reducing the outbursts of acne. Fatty acids have been proven to be an effective anti-inflammatory, and they are abundant in fishes. Although research is ongoing on keto diets and its benefits, it has been established that the keto diet is essential for clearer, improved, and radiant skin.

5. Keto and Anti-Aging

Naturally, aging comes with many diseases. Although there is no study on the effect of a keto diet on human brain cells, studies on mice proved that brain cells improve when on a keto diet.

Many scientific studies have shown that the keto diet has positive effects on people suffering from Alzheimer's disease. It is recognized that diets with a good proportion of good nutrients, healthy fats, low carbohydrate, high protein content, low sugar content, and also abundant in antioxidants help to improve our well-being while these diets also shield us from harmful substances from poor diets.

Research has also proven that an efficient way of slowing down the aging process is by consuming more fatty acids which the body converts to energy rather than heavy reliance on sugar as the primary energy source.

Also, the consumption of a moderate quantity of calories and eating less is one of the basic health principles which help to reduce our susceptibility to obesity and its consequences.

Although studies on keto diets are relatively small, however, the few but thrilling benefits derived from ketogenic diet on our well-being emphasizes the effectiveness of the diet in aiding natural growth while keeping the natural effects of aging in check. A regular western diet with high sugar content and processed foods are not suitable for easy aging process.

6. **Keto and Hunger**

One of the reasons that many people avoid dieting is because many traditional diets make people feel hungry, allowing them to feel deprived, which makes them easily give up. However, due to its low carbohydrate and low-calorie content, the keto diet plugs this gap, which makes people feel filled and happy.

7. **Keto and Eyesight**

It is known that high blood sugar levels increase the likelihood of cataracts developing. Keto diets help keep good eyesight and also protect against cataracts due to their effective control of the body sugar level.

8. **Keto and Autism**

Although keto diets increase the brain's flexibility, a recent study of hungry autistic patients has shown that the keto diet actually deals with autism. The study, which showed positive effects of keto diets on autism, revealed that students exhibited improved autistic behavior, especially those with lower autism.

Macronutrients and Micronutrients

The benefits of a ketogenic diet, as mentioned earlier, are not limited to weight loss, but the diet comes with a range of health benefits. The positive reviews for the aforementioned diet have increased significantly, and this rise in popularity has prompted researchers and scientists to perform additional controlled trials to test its long-term effectiveness. The primary reason this diet helps in weight loss is the decreased appetite, which naturally makes keeping the low calorie intake quite easy. If you over-consume calories, no matter the quality of your macronutrients, it will inhibit weight loss in your body.

A macronutrient's mass and ratio define how much one can consume of the macronutrient. Based on the diet regimen the amount of each macronutrient in low-carb diets will differ. The macronutrient composition is as follows when it comes to ketogenic diet, macronutrient composition= 5 percent carbs + 15 percent protein + 80 percent fats.

A traditional ketogenic diet needs you to eat 20 to 30 g of carbs in a day while fat intake depends on protein and carbs intake. A few examples of macronutrient-rich foods are:

- Fats (coconut oil, olive oil, macadamia nuts, avocado, brazil nuts)
- Protein (eggs, cheese, yogurt, milk, chicken, fish)

- Carbohydrates (sweets, sugary snacks, bread, cereals, pasta, potatoes)

Carbohydrates

The dietary carbohydrates also called carbs are responsible for energy generation in your body. The human body uses the carbohydrates to generate energy. Experts say however that carbs are not the main energy source. The body can make energy out of the dietary fat and protein.

When you follow a ketogenic diet, the carb intake is extremely low, which is a complete contrast to the current western diet. People who follow the modern western diet today derive their dietary calories from the carbs they eat. Your body releases insulin when you consume carbohydrates and this in turn hinders the production of ketones in the liver making it impossible for the body to get into ketosis. Therefore, when you are on a keto diet, it's important to monitor and control your carb intake. A standard keto diet recommends reducing your carb intake to or below 5 per cent.

A properly planned and well-designed ketogenic diet will have fiber intake along with fats as the crucial component. Fiber is important for keeping your gut health and keeping you satiated as it increases the bulk of the food. Including fiber-rich cruciferous vegetables and leafy greens is crucial for a proper ketogenic diet. The total carbohydrates minus the total fiber will be your net carb consumption, and it is this measure that will help you track your carb intake.

You need to understand that an increase in fiber intake does not affect blood ketone levels and blood glucose levels as well. Fibers are immune to digestion, which can provide you with a satiated sensation that reduces your appetite.

Proteins

Proteins are large molecular structures that consist of long and tiny amino acid chains. What are Dietary Protein Functions? They are responsible for:

- Glucose conversion through gluconeogenesis
- Charging the intermediates in different metabolic pathways such as the Krebs Cycle
- Building the functional and structural components of the cells

Although the body can use protein as a source of energy, that is not its primary function. Hence, it is important to have an adequate protein balance in your body to maintain the muscle mass while following the keto diet. You must ensure that the calories from protein intake do not exceed 20 to 25 percent or else the protein gluconeogenesis process may hinder ketone production.

Let your protein intake be somewhere between 0.8 to 1.2 g per kilogram of your body weight when you begin with the ketogenic diet. This can help you balance your protein requirements against the potential for unnecessary gluconeogenesis.

Fats

Obesity has always been at the spotlight on the wrong side. Many people have confused this with being the reason for increased weight and heart problems. Fat is the only macronutrient possessing molecules of triglycerides. The main functionality of fat as a nutrition in your food is to provide you with additional levels of energy and make up your system's key structural and functional parts.

Nutrient fat is often confused with fat. The fat in your cells and the different types of available fat molecules are not identical.

The different types of fat molecules are:

- Adipocytes (Individual cells that contain the lipids or fats)

- Adipose tissue (the tissue that store the energy inside the adipocytes as lipid droplets or fats). This is body fat)
- Fatty acids (Molecules made up of carbon atomic chains bonded together with carboxylic acid at one end)
- Lipids (a generic term used for polar and insoluble biological fat molecules. We have various lipid type molecules like phospholipids, mono-, di-and triglycerols, and cholesterols)
- Triglycerides (a lipid molecule made up of glycerol a cholesterol).

Such lipids, once digested, migrate as fatty acids and triglycerides through the bloodstream. The body either uses lipids for energy production or retains them in the adipose tissue. Dietary fat is the fat you consume whilst stored body fat is the fat (calories) stored as a reserve by the body. Triglycerides are the most important energy in a ketogenic diet, where they account for more than 70 per cent of the dietary calories.

Fatty acids can be saturated or unsaturated—a saturated fatty acid will have no double carbon bonds while an unsaturated fatty acid will have one or more double carbon bonds. Saturated fats like coconut oil, butter, etc. are stable, and can be at room temperature in their solid state. During the earlier days, dietary unsaturated fats have led to the development of high blood pressure and heart disease, thus either prohibiting or limiting the intake of such fats.

Unsaturated fatty acids can be divided as follows:

- Monounsaturated fats (it has only one double carbon bond)
- Polyunsaturated fats (it has multiple double carbon bonds)

The fatty acid behavior is determined by the number of double bonds it holds. At room temperature, these fatty acids are mostly in liquid state (example: olive oil). Initially, people believed that unsaturated fats were healthier than saturated fats but experts say saturated fats are healthy fats. Through intake of monounsaturated and polyunsaturated fats the blood biomarkers (lower blood triglycerides) boost. When taking a keto diet, it is crucial that you eat sufficient unsaturated fats. A rise in fat intake is not causing cardiovascular problems.

Your body metabolizes the fats according to the chain length. The body absorbs and moves the long-chain fatty acids to the lymphatic drainage channel, after which the fatty acids pass into the bloodstream. But with short-chain fatty acids and medium-chain fatty acids, that doesn't happen. They do not enter the lymph system but travel directly from the intestine through the bloodstream to the liver. If you deliver massive amounts of these short-chain and medium-chain fatty acids to the liver at once, converting those fatty acids into ketone bodies can trigger the liver.

Medium chain fatty acids are highly ketogenic in coconut oil. But if a few people consume a large amount of medium-chain fatty acids, they may have an upset stomach. So those people won't be able to artificially raise their ketone levels. Once you summarize all of these definitions, you will be able to understand that to induce ketosis, you need to increase your dietary fat intake to a limit. Make sure you include a variety of healthy fat from different plant sources : almonds, coconut oil, avocados, olive oil, etc.

The micronutrients, on the opposite, are equally important and must be obtained in minimum quality from the diet. Vitamins and minerals are common examples of micronutrients.

Micronutrients in a Keto diet

During a keto diet, salt, magnesium, potassium and calcium are the essential micronutrients that should go into the body. For the following reasons, you need to be aware of your micronutrient intake:

- If you reduce your carb intake, you may need to lower the consumption of various other micronutrient-rich foods. Example: Vegetables and fruit

- A few nutrients (sodium, magnesium, potassium, calcium) may go off-balance in your body during the initial 28 days of your keto diet, as most of these nutrients go out of your body as urine or sweat increases, and the frequency of excretion. Your body naturally resolves the problem after it's adapted to the diet.

- You should increase your sodium intake, as more extracellular fluid is lost due to frequent urination. Sodium's core functionality is to maintain the potential for water balance, blood volume, and cell membrane. It is also essential for the conduction of nerves and for acid-base balance.

Your sodium levels may show a slight dip during the initial stages of the keto diet and so it is important that you add extra sodium to your meals by adding more salt. This may also that the keto diet's common side effect-muscle cramps often associated with low sodium.

Potassium's fundamental functionality is mostly associated with:

- Electrical activity in cells (cardiomyocytes and neurons)
- Cell membrane potential.

As with sodium, potassium levels often dropped due to increased excretion, so you need to add more dark green foods, avocados, and nuts to your keto diet.

Another important element is Magnesium, which plays a major role in the function of the immune, nerve, and muscle. Magnesium levels dropped as a result of increased excretion at the start of keto diet.

On a keto diet you rarely encounter a calcium deficiency because the daily consumption of leafy greens, cheese and various similar foods will hold your calcium in order. Calcium is essential for your bone health, muscle contraction and cardiovascular wellbeing

What are Ketones?

So, what exactly do these ketones come from and where? As mentioned above, when your body exhausts its reserves of glucose (glycogen) it will be looking for another alternative source of energy. This is when it gets digging into the fat storehouse of the body because stored fat will help fuel the cells with the energy required.

Since there is no glucose in the body, the stored fats will be taken in by your liver and converted to fatty acids. These fatty acids then split into functional compounds known as ketone bodies (known as ketones). Your body uses those ketones to give your body cells and brain cells electricity. The best part is when blood ketone levels increase reducing the appetite. The explanation for increased strength is because the brain requires another source of energy to generate.

Your liver develops three distinct types of ketone bodies:

- Acetoacetate
- Beta-Hydroxybutryate
- Acetone

Your body can fuel itself from ketones in two different ways:

- Your body can make its own ketones by fasting or by increasing your fat intake and reducing your carb intake by forcing glucose abstinence
- You can also feed your body with actual ketones by consuming exogenous ketones (ketone supplements)

When your body is on a ketogenic diet, it acts as a fat-burning machine. This naturally leads to low insulin levels and the power to burn fat increases as it becomes easy to access the fat stores. When it produces ketones, your body is in ketosis, and the fastest way to shift your body to ketosis is to fast. But for ever fasting is impossible, and this has led to the development of the ketogenic diet.

Is it possible to lose weight because the body enters into ketosis?

Once your body starts eating fat contained in ketones, your body changes to ketosis. But why is that going to bring me down weight? I understand from whence you come. Let me just give you an example of this.

Just imagine you've stored a pile of coal for the winter ahead. When it's winter, some of these piles of coal are scooped up for heat into the furnace. The pile gets smaller as you continue to use up all the coal. Likewise, your body burns the stored fat in your body in ketosis and as it continues to make use of the accumulated fats (which is the extra flab, water weight, excess calories, etc.), you become lighter, i.e. you reduce weight. Here the coal is the stored fat and your energy is the heat you receive in winter.

There are numerous studies on how a well-planned ketogenic diet has helped countless people lose weight by improving their health markers and improving their overall health condition. Thermodynamics is another significant reason to lose weight on the ketogenic diet! You get rid of one big macronutrient-carbohydrates-when you follow the keto diet!

The following list includes the carbohydrate rich food items:

- Soda
- Bagels
- Fruit smoothies
- Bread
- Sugar candies
- White rice
- Pasta

These foods have a high caloric value, and those carbs are stored as fat in your body when you over-eat. When these carb-rich foods are restricted or eliminated, you consume fewer calories. You loose weight when you burn more calories than you consume. This is one of the main reasons why most calorie-restricted diets cause weight loss when done correctly regardless of the proportion of the food you eat. You don't focus on the body composition, food quality or muscle synthesis on this type of diet but it's more about the amount of food consumed (smaller portions of food).

When your body is adapted to the keto routine, you feel satiated with fewer calories, resulting in faster and easier weight loss in the end. Yet note, you'll probably gain more weight if you overeat on a keto diet. So, don't expect to lose weight regularly after eating 6000 calories of bacon, beef and butter! You need to learn how to eat healthy!

The ketogenic diet assists in weight loss as well as helps in:

- Epilepsy treatment
- Type 2 diabetes
- Managing PCOS (Polycystic ovary syndrome)
- Treats acne
- Showing improvement in neurological diseases such as MS (multiple sclerosis and Parkinson's)
- Reducing the risk of cardiovascular and respiratory diseases

Researchers are doing more research to understand how the keto diet impacts Alzheimer's patients and similar health problems.

Side-effects of the Ketogenic diet

You'll feel weak and exhausted for the initial two to three days when you start with the keto diet, because your blood glucose levels are low. Either your body has yet to enter ketosis mode, or the production of ketones has not reached a stage where it can provide your brain and body with enough fuel. This particular state of your body will result in a number of possible side effects. These side effects lead to keto flu and the symptoms common are:

- Fatigue
- Headache
- Muscle cramps
- Dizziness
- Nausea

If the food you eat does not provide the required amount of macronutrients and micronutrients to your body, you tend to develop other symptoms that are ahead of keto flu.

Some other symptoms people experience after the adjustment period are:

- Hair loss
- Constipation

- Elevated cholesterol levels
- Increase in blood triglycerides
- Bad breath
- Gallstones
- Exhaustion and tiredness that makes it difficult to maintain your physical performance

You will need to provide adequate micronutrients and calories to your body to overcome those symptoms. If you reduce the consumption of vegetables and fruits in a keto diet due to the high carb content, you do not consume enough fiber content which contributes to vitamin deficiency. The keto diet can also change the way the kidneys function-they can excrete more electrolytes like sodium and potassium. In such cases, you must include supplements to reduce the electrolyte imbalance in your body.

If your carb intake is extremely low, your keto diet is more effective–a stringent keto diet would want you to eat less than 20 grams of net carbs a day.

WHAT IS CHAFFLES?

The basic recipe for a chaffle includes cheddar cheese, almond flour and an ointment. In a pot, you mix the ingredients together, and spill it over the waffle maker. Waffle makers are possibly on the rise right now, after the other day this recipe for the chaffle exploded. Make sure the waffle maker is sprayed really well. The waffle turned out great, and the outside was crispy and the middle was fluffy.

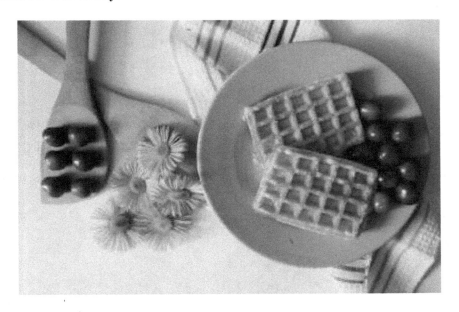

HOW TO MAKE CHAFFLES

What do I need to make a chaffle?

- 1 large egg
- 1/2 c. Cheddar – I used Happy Farms brand from Aldi
- 2 tablespoons of almond flour

Preparation

- Preheat your waffle maker when preheating is needed.
- Whisk the potato, cheddar and almond flour together in a cup, until well combined.
- Spray the cooking spray on the waffle maker and pour the caffle batter over the waffle maker. Close to prepare for 3 to 4 minutes of waffle. My waffle maker is set to its own automatic timer.
- Take the waffle iron, and enjoy it.

THE EFFECT WHEN KETO MEETS CHAFFLES

A distinguished surgeon at the Mayo Clinic advised in 1921 to pursue what he called a ketogenic weight-reduction strategy, an excessive-fat diet intended to be so carbohydrate-poor that it could practically imitate the state of fasting. He says: We had intervals of hunger back in our hunter-gatherer days, the place our bodies needed to adapt to the lack of meals by breaking down our protein and fat stores into sources of fuel. Carb cycling is simply anytime the daily keto-consuming routine adds a healthier carb-day. Preserve studying for the small print, plus study on this weight reduction plan which meals you may eat on.

And some early analysis suggests it may have implications for regulating blood sugar in people with diabetes. As a vegetarian, living low-carb and keto might be typically difficult. Fresh meat and poultry, together with potassium, selenium and zinc, contain no carbs, and are rich in B vitamins and a number of other minerals. The ketogenic diet regimen, or keto weight loss program, is a particular type of low carb weight reduction strategy based on a certain ratio of macronutrients, or macros, with a goal of reaching a state called ketosis.

The Keto diet ignores the proven fact that the ingested excess fat leads to the adsorption of drastically increased amounts of highly poisonous lipophiles similar to TCDD, PCBs and chlorinated pesticides. If you include a cheat day, as a result of water retention, you may feel like you're piling on the weight. With all the wellbeing benefits, the Ketogenic weight loss plan is absolutely defined.

In case you eat at the same time each day, we recommend using both repeatable alerts in the iPhone Clock app or iPhone Reminders for pre-meal reviews. Initially developed for the treatment of extreme epilepsy in infants and adolescents under medical supervision, as we speak the ketogenic dietary regimen shifts to the mainstream as a low-carbohydrate weight reduction software and as a means of reducing cardiometabolic hazard components— but not without controversy.

Keto naturally lowers blood sugar ranges because of the type of meal you are eating. Consider eating only a small portion of a banana and slicing it very finely, or combining bananas with banana-flavored extracts as a supplement, for those who try keto and enjoy bananas. Unfortunately, the general public was not necessarily exposed to the reality of dietary ketosis, and as a result, they do not consider that being in it is a healthy state.

Our ketogenic cookbooks make low-carb eating simple and scrumptious, from the satiating fat-fuelled breakfasts to the finest sugar-free desserts. To mitigate this, you can aim for the first few weeks of a routine low-carb diet regimen. Changing to a ketogenic weight-loss plan could lead to changes in constipation-like bowel habits.

The simple truth is that the consumption of carbs is causing blood sugar to rise. The right way to quantify the macronutrient ratios and percentages for a traditional ketogenic weight loss program exists in great debate. In case you increase your protein intake, your physique could burn protein as fuel instead of fats (a process called gluconeogenesis). Fat bombs such as unsweetened chocolate or coconut oil can help people achieve their daily fat intake targets.

During ketosis, the liver converts our bodies or ketones into fatty acids into ketones. These by-products turn into the new supply of energy for your body. When you turn to a ketogenic diet it is natural to feel changes in your pores and skin. Because of the ketogenic weight loss program, there are many variations— many of which are marketed by fitness blogs in celebrity circles, trend magazines, and online — there is some confusion about the eating form.

Keto flu is a period of time which refers back to the period after you start the diet when your body is changing for power to burn fat. How it works: Usually no sugar, caffeine, prostatricum pareri grains, legumes, milk or treats are permitted for 30 days. In a six-month experimental & clinical cardiology research involving 83 obese adults, those on the keto food plan misplaced an average of

33 kilos, while reducing their dangerous (LDL) cholesterol levels and increasing their good (HDL) ldl cholesterol levels.

Depending on the Ladies ' Institute's Dr. Laurie Cullen, as MCTs are ingested into the bloodstream, they skip the course of absorption of the longer chain fat. Low-carb diets have been discovered to cause no damage to the liver of healthy people in studies conducted to investigate the short-term effects. Keto smoothies: To make this breakfast staple you can see lots of low-carb recipes.

The ketogenic food plan is only right for you if you are diligent, as sustaining the ketosis state requires disciplined counting of carbohydrates. Low-carb recipes usually have less than 15 g of carbs per serving, and really low-carb recipes have less than 5 g of carbs per serving, making them especially suitable for keto diets. When the body is in the state of ketosis, ketones are produced which are created by the breakdown of the fat which may be present in the liver.

Research have shown people who eat more refined grains gain more weight over time, "says McKeown. The keto weight loss plan is a weight loss program that's safe and most people can really feel good about trying it out. Word: In keto, the allotments of sugar, fats, proteins, and calories are expressed in grams each day and are considered macros. In those on ketogenic diets inadequate intake of 17 micronutrients has been reported.

Keto breath usually goes away after a short period of time when the fats are adapted to your physique. CaloriesDRIis an average daily Dietary Reference calories based on age, class, weight, peak and level of personal activity. Under keto, the levels of insulin (the hormone-storing fats) drop dramatically, which turns the body into a burning engine for fats. Start your usual ketogenic Caloric stage and macro-nutrient ratio once more after the second 24-hour carb-load period.

It also converts fat into ketones within the liver and might provide this energy to the brain. Still, many people (especially women) have difficulty getting enough protein on a daily basis. Using our keto foods pointers and visible guides will make estimating roughly how many carbs you eat in a day easy. 5-10 per cent of carbohydrates calories. That's right, your metabolism is not stoked "throughout the day by consuming small meals or grazing.

Food is important for helping your digestion and regular body features, and low carb diets such as keto have a diuretic effect on your physique. Keto compliant diet checklist Huge. A cup of cooked whole-wheat noodles has about forty-one internet carbs that would blow into a single small portion of my daily carb allowance. This can help your physique adapt to such changes and burn more fats earlier than you can completely remove carbs throughout the ketogenic weight loss programme.

It's also related to a variety of ongoing illnesses. It is estimated that about 300,000 people die each year from weight-related diseases in the United States alone. Completely different approaches for weight reduction using decreased calorie and fat consumption in conjunction with train have failed to show consistent long-term performance. Current research from various laboratories, along with our own, has shown that a wealthy excessive fat weight-reduction plan in polyunsaturated fatty acids (ketogenic dietary regimen) is quite effective in reducing body weight and the risk elements for various chronic conditions.

Although ketosis in our modern instances is not necessarily required for survival, this particular metabolic condition is likely to have some advantages. Zhao Z, Lange DJ, Youtianiouk A, MacGrogan D, Ho L, Suh J, Humala N, Thiyagarajan M, Wang J, Pasinetti GM. A ketogenic diet as a potential experimental medical treatment for lateral amyotrophic sclerosis. Yet she claims it could be risky to go keto with a lot of saturated fats and that patient "cholesterols can just go nuts" on the diet.

TRF is the practice of reducing the feeding period from 4–10 hours throughout the day to some spot, and fasting the rest of the time. In practice, a keto weight-reduction diet is rather straightforward (low carbohydrates, excess fat, mild protein). A: As long as you eat enough protein and energy, your muscle tissue won't go anywhere just because you're scaling back on your carb consumption.

Before you lose fats, you don't have to use all of your power stores, as on a typical high-carb weight reduction plan. It has been shown that keto diets help improve cholesterol levels. Protein is part of the keto food plan, but sometimes it does not differentiate between lean protein meals and protein sources rich in beef, pork, and bacon-reminiscent saturated fats.

Cyclic ketogenic weight loss program (CKD): This diet includes intervals of higher-carb refeeds, similar to 5 ketogenic days of 2 high-carb days adopted. It is very important to remember that there are completely different conditions and people and that no one weight loss weight loss plan suits all. Anyone following a Ketogenic diet, however, try to keep in ketosis for as long as possible— usually weeks or even months at a time.

When you focus on day by day measuring, you'll find that your weight fluctuates with your high and low carb days. Kielb S, Koo HP, Bloom DA, Faerber GJ. Nephrolithiasis on ketogenic dietary regimen. Easy carbohydrate consisting of refined flour and added sugar transforms easily into blood sugar (glucose) when you consume it. In case you think that the ketogenic food plan is all about safe dwelling for a second now, you might perceive.

It can often be a motivating and useful indicator of the transition occurring in your physique to realize those quantities and see how they enhance or decrease relying on what you consume daily. This makes it a very good eating regimen to observe if you plan to add a weight-lifting regimen to your lifestyle, if you are trying to stabilize blood sugar levels and if you might want to increase your ldl cholesterol numbers.

If you happen to be serious about losing a few pounds and need to create a new lifestyle for yourself then the problem of 28-Day Weight Loss is for you. If your ketone test results show that after drinking this a lot for a whole week you are not in ketosis, then decrease your intake by as much as 20 g per day. The excessive consumption of fats on this eating regimen feeds your brain and body positively for hours without getting hungry.

Vizthum notes that these attempts at the keto weight loss program would make an honest effort to consume entire meals and not turn to processed foods that might be legal, but are not wholesome in any other situation (yes, this includes keto fast food options). In addition to better health-based benefits, this can guarantee any weight-loss result.

The 1:1 diet scheme is much more versatile than other weight loss schemes, and it is the ONLY scheme that gives you committed, one-to - one help from your own personal weight reduction strategy guide. Taking a high blood pressure remedy and using a low-carb dietary regimen can put you at risk of low blood pressure within a matter of days, so consulting your GP in learning how to handle this might be clever before you start.

For additional data, take a look at this text about the effects of low-carb diets for diabetes patients. A limited amount of carbohydrate intake will move the body to burning ketones as your primary fuel supply. Once parents apply the medical information of the infant, our team takes the view that it is fastidious to decide whether a ketogenic weight loss plan is an appropriate therapy and which approach can be the best for each baby.

Besides that, the diet is also great for people living with diabetes. Shut up monitoring of blood ketones and blood glucose levels will occur throughout admission. You just track the carbohydrates as a supplement by observing labels and trying to stay inside a product depending on 30 g of net carbs per day (or 50 g of general carbs). If you're running out of time and have to stop at a fast-food restaurant, take a look at our Keto Fast Meals Listing This low-carb quick-food meal guide gives you our favorite fast-food restaurants to eat at, along with what fast-food options we would get.

The Johns Hopkins clinical epilepsy program has over a hundred years of experience in treating epilepsy with the ketogenic dietary regimen. Although on a ketogenic diet regimen you will eat bacon, the remainder of the continuum is proscribed.

Nonetheless, they know simple methods to make fats and protein look scrumptious, and how to help you manage your shopping and meal planning routines For this and any other dietary modification, any steering is beneficial.

As with hunger, going into ketosis usually takes some time like soon as we stop eating carbohydrates. For some, the keto food plan may be easier to maintain than other diets as you get to consume scrumptious foods such as almonds, avocados and cheese, while feeling full still. Every day, you make an attempt to eat less than 20-50 grams of internet carbohydrates, to make the weight loss program 70 percent fats.

Once you get on the keto path, you'll realize it's more than just another fashionable, consumer plan. In addition, there are numbers of ZERO calories and ample opportunities to stack on fats and some protein for higher beneficial muscle properties. Many individuals discover that following a Paleo dietary regimen, the bowel health and weight loss could be supported. This in flip forces the body to convert fats into power, forming ketones that could be released from the liver.

Anecdotally, they feel satiated on fewer calories as soon as some people turn into keto-adapted —which ends in easier weight loss. The underlying theory of ketogenic weight loss is that without getting thirsty you will help you be in a state of caloric restriction. New Atkins weight reduction program (MAD)–A modified version of Atkins used to treat epilepsy, MAD is less stringent than traditional keto, allowing for greater protein and fat quantities.

If you need to calculate your "macros" when you first start a ketogenic weight reduction plan, I use this one Your ratios must be closed to 5 percent carbs, 20-25 percent protein and 70-75 percent fat. But if keto ends up being a food regimen in which you may be able to continue happily and comfortably, and it works for you, then it may be worth your time. Hence, the emphasis on a low carb weight reduction strategy with high fat.

The less calories you eat, the better it seems to be for weight reduction, suppression of appetite, type 2 diabetes and more. It's about discovering the recipes that you're keen on is perfect for your physique. Because of this fact, the present examination confirms that a ketogenic weight loss program is safe to use for a longer time frame than previously shown.

Ketogenic Weight Loss Plan: Jamie Ken Moore's Step by Step Guide For Newbies does just that, breaking down the fundamentals of keto in an entertainer-friendly guidebook. While most people finally change to ketosis, if you don't keep low enough carbohydrate ranges, your body may go in and out of the state of fat burning. If you're in ketosis, some may experience ramped weight loss and increased body capacity, reduced sugar levels, higher mind working, and other awesomeness for others.

You may still get the benefits of ketosis, while eating an assorted and balanced weight loss program through intermittent fasting, "Dr. Ring says. The ketogenic food plan is about making your physique transition into ketosis, which is a physiological process in which you continue using fat stores as an alternative to glycogen for power. Dietary ketosis in mild cognitive impairment increases memory.

KETO DIET AND CANCER

Cancer has become a deadly disease in our societies in recent years. While cancer was around before the 20th century, it was less pronounced then than now. Indeed, our daily activities and dietary principles have increased our cancer exposure, making it a major threat to human life. Yes, it has been estimated that nearly 1,600 Americans suffer daily from cancer. It shows that our bodies are not responding well to daily pollutant or toxin exposures.

Although disclosing any case of cancer to doctors and other relevant medical providers is very significant, it is interesting to address the vital role keto diets play in cancer treatment. The fat content in the diet would be as high as 90 percent when using keto diet to fight cancer. This is primarily because cancer cells feed on carbohydrates and growth sugar; thus, reducing carbohydrates to a minimum level makes it difficult for cancer cells to grow or develop in the body system. Basically, the keto diet reduces the availability of carbohydrates for the development of the cancer cells, which ultimately leads to the death of the cancer cells or drastic reduction in their growth potentials.

Another way keto diet helps to reduce cancer is that to develop energy, cancer cells need calories. Keto diets reduce the number of calories present in the body system, resulting in less food supply needed to grow cancer cells. Insulin is also needed for tumor cell growth. The growth of tumor cells is severely reduced by reducing the insulin level in the body.

Keto diet also helps provide the body with ketones that are used as energy sources in the body system. Ketones, on the other hand, cause cancer cells to grow at a very slow pace, thus helping to reduce body sizes and cancer cell growth.

Also, the keto diet helps to prevent the development of cancer cells in people with diabetes. Diabetic patients are usually susceptible to cancer because of their high blood sugar levels; however, keto diet, which is effective in lowering blood sugar levels, helps reduce cancer cell growth. As a result, their exposure to cancer development is limited.

Results of past research studies have indicated that ketogenic diets help in treating cancer by:

- Halting the development of cancer cells.

- Providing the body with healthy cells after eliminating cancerous cells.
- Altering the digestive system of the body and helping the body to deny cancer cells of the nutrients needed for growth.
- Reducing the level of insulin in the body system which prevents the inception and growth of cancer cells.

Foods to Eat

It's important to start your diet with all natural, single-ingredient foods. You can add one or all of the following items to your keto food list.

Vegetables that grow above the ground

You are free to use either fresh veggies or the frozen ones when you include vegetables in your diet recipes. On a keto diet, the best way to get some good fat into your body is by getting vegetables – those that rise above the ground. You can choose which one;

All the leafy green vegetables

- Cauliflower
- Broccoli

- Cabbage
- Zucchini
- Avocado
- Bell peppers
- Mushrooms
- Asparagus
- Peas
- Beans (Green, black)
- Tomatoes
- Lettuce
- Kale
- Cucumber
- Brussels Sprouts
- Celery
- Eggplant
- Artichokes

You can use olive oil or coconut oil or butter to cook the vegetables and allow more healthy fats to get into your system. When preparing a vegetable salad, you may dress with olive oil. Veggies are your best fat delivery system that can add to your keto diet meals more flavor, color and variety.

Upon your keto diet you will end up eating more vegetables as you will need to replace your rice, potatoes and pasta with mixed vegetables.

Other Vegetables

You can also include other vegetables such as:

- Onions
- Garlic
- Ginger
- Radish
- Turnip

Healthy Fats

Avocados, beans, and nuts are the essential food products high in healthy fats. Use less cashews when choosing nuts, since they are high in carbs. Just go in for it:

- Pecan nuts
- Macadamia nuts
- Almonds
- Brazil nuts
- Walnuts

Nut butters may also be added to your food list. But you need to be a little vigilant when snacking on almonds, because you tend to eat more than you need to feel satiated.

Seeds are good sources of healthy fats, as well. Include plenty of seeds in your keto recipes:

- Pumpkin seeds
- Pistachios
- Chia seeds
- Flaxseeds

Healthy oils are a great source of fat for your body:

- Coconut oil
- Olive oil
- Avocado oil

Fruit

You can include a moderate amount of berries to your keto diet:

- Strawberry
- Blackberry
- Raspberry

Blueberries have more carbohydrates so be patient when using them-sometimes use one or two.

Some other fruits you might choose to include in your keto diet are:

- Plum
- Cherries
- Peach
- Mandarin
- Cantaloupe
- Kiwi
- Lemon
- Coconut (the white fleshy thing – the meat of the coconut)

Meatless Proteins

When you decide on a completely vegetarian or vegan keto diet, the following meatless choices may be included:

- Seitan
- Tempeh
- Tofu

Condiments

You can include the following condiments to your keto diet plan:

- Pepper
- Herbs
- Salt
- Spices
- Horseradish
- Aioli

Meat

The processed meats should be avoided. You must choose unprocessed meats because they are mostly keto-friendly and contain fewer carbs. If you'd like to go for the healthiest choice, consider grass-fed and organic beef. But since keto diet is high in fat and not protein, you don't need to add enormous amounts of meat to your diet.

When you eat more meat than you end up with extra fat, which is more than the body needs. This will force the body out of ketosis as the cycle of gluconeogenesis-turning your proteins into glucose-takes place. So a small to moderate amount of meat is more than appropriate for you to adhere to your ketogenic eating regimen.

It is better to avoid cold cuts, meatballs and sausages since all these processed meats also contain additional carbohydrates which are not good for your body. When you buy processed meat always look for the ingredients (if you have no other choice). Note, the consumption of carb must be less than 5 per cent.

You need to be careful with how much of the following meats you consume:

- White meat
- Turkey
- Chicken

Pork products

- Ham
- Sausage
- Bacon

Red meat

- Steak

Fatty meats are good for keto diets.

Seafood and Fish

Fatty fish are excellent choices for a good ketogenic diet:

- Tuna
- Salmon
- Mackerel
- Trout

Also other seafood like shellfish are a good choice for your keto diet.

Eggs

You can eat them in any form:

- Boiled eggs
- Scrambled eggs
- Omelets
- Fried eggs (with coconut oil or butter)

If you buy eggs, go for eggs that are omega-3, pastured or free-range (eggs that come from animals that are free-range). Always opt for the organic alternative! You shouldn't eat more than 36 eggs per day given the cholesterol level in the eggs. But if you're allowed to eat fewer eggs, good for you! Try adding as much unprocessed cheese and butter as possible when you are making keto-friendly egg recipes. Sticking to the cream, cheddar or mozzarella cheese is safer.

High-fat Sauces, Natural Fat

When mentioned earlier, most of your calories would come from fat when you are on a keto diet and so it is crucial that you choose the natural source of fat. Eggs, meat, fish and seafood are fat-rich foods, but by cooking in coconut fat, olive oil, coconut oil, butter, etc., it is also important that you add more fat to your dishes. You can also include keto-friendly high-fat sauces, wraps, and spreads such as:

- Garlic butter
- Béarnaise sauce
- Yellow mustard
- Dijon mustard
- Sriracha mayonnaise
- Full-fat mayonnaise
- Buffalo hot sauce
- Creamy salad dressings

- Pesto
- Alfredo sauce
- Chimichurri
- Nacho cheese sauce
- Tzatziki
- Low-sugar BBQ sauce
- Guacamole
- Herbed butter

High-fat dairy products

Until now, when you're shopping on your weekly grocery shopping, you've seen people going for low-fat cheese, low-fat butter etc. You'll have to go for the opposite in your case, though! The keto diet allows you to add as many high-fat nutritious products as possible, and high-fat dairy is one inexpensive option. Can you include:

- Heavy cream (for cooking)
- Grass-fed cream and butter
- High-fat unprocessed cheese
- Cheddar
- Mozzarella
- Blue
- Goats cheese (optional)

- High-fat yogurts (don't over-eat)

In your coffee, you can use milk sparingly, as the milk sugar will add up to your carb. No Latte café, sorry! If you're not hungry, don't snack too much on cheese as it might delay your weight-loss program.

Drinks that are allowed

Water is everybody's first choice regardless of whether you survive or not. To keep your body hydrated you need to drink a sufficient amount of water. A well hydrated body with no hiccups will do its best! You can have it back to the keto diet:

- Plain water
- Sparkling water
- Iced water
- Hot water
- Natural flavored water (adding limes, sliced cucumbers or lemons to your water)
- Salted water (add half to one teaspoon of salt to your drinking water if you are suffering from keto flu symptoms or headaches)

If you don't add sugar, cream or milk to it, you should drink Coffee. But if you're not used to black coffee, you can add some cream, or some milk. You can also throw in coconut oil and butter to make your coffee into a fat-energized cup. You too have the option of bulletproof coffee! And don't forget to cut back on your coffee cream, fat or milk if you feel a lag in your weight-loss schedule.

Tea is another good option in a keto diet but here too there is no sugar again. You can go for the tea choices below:

- Herbal tea
- Black tea
- Green tea
- Mint tea
- Orange Pekoe tea

The bone broth is another beverage you can eat on the keto diet. Not only is this drink satiating but it's also full of electrolytes and nutrients that can keep your body hydrated for hours. It is easy to make and you can add some coconut oil or butter to it, because the extra energy quotient Vegetable stock is similar to your bone broth as well. You can make a simple and nutritious stock from mixed vegetables (for the extra bit of taste, add more onions and garlic).

Foods to Eat in Moderation

- Have one serving of root vegetables, such as yams, parsnip, carrots, and turnips per day.
- Fruits should be taken once a day due to the high contents of sugar in them.
- A glass of dry wine, vodka, whiskey, and brandy once a week. And cocktails with sugar should be avoided.
- A little portion of chocolate with cocoa contents of 75 percent or higher once a week.

Foods to Avoid

- Any food with a substantial amount of sugar content, including cereals, soft drinks, juices, and sports drinks, candies, and chocolate. Artificial sweeteners or ingredients should be avoided.
- Foods with high starch contents such as pasta and potatoes, bread, potato chips, and French fries, cooking oils, and margarine.
- All varieties of beers.

KETO DIET AND EPILEPSY

It may be interesting to note that the keto diet was primarily intended to treat epilepsy rather than the weight loss or diabetes treatment it is known for. In 1924, Keto diet was designed by a doctor to assist his patients with epilepsy.

Epilepsy is a nervous system disorder that causes frequent seizures at any point in the human body. Typical epilepsy signs involve hallucinations, spasms, but it can also cause a rare psychological view of the world. The symptoms are caused by abnormal activity in many of the cases, and the severity of the symptoms varies among people. Anyone may suffer seizures, but only those with more than two seizures in a day are diagnosed as epileptic. More importantly, convulsions are more common among the young due to their brain still being in the developmental stage. While seizures can be managed by drugs, medications are not always effective in managing seizures.

In 1924, Dr. Russell Wilder of the Mayo Clinic performed great research that gave birth to keto diet. Research shows that ketogenic diet is very effective for children diagnosed with epilepsy. It was then embraced by other medical practitioners until the emergence of new medications that could cure seizures as they prefer drug prescriptions to diet recommendations.

Meanwhile, those who prefer keto diets have seen remarkable improvements in their wellness as they experience a drastic reduction in seizures. Ironically, doctors are now embracing the recommendation of high fats and low carbohydrates diet to treat their patients, and this has proven to be effective.

The study in the Journal of Pediatrics, which was published in 1998, also reinforced the effectiveness of keto diets in curing seizures. It was reported that 150 children suffering from seizures continued experiencing seizures despite the anti-seizure medications provided for them. However, the children were placed on ketogenic diets, and their progress was carefully examined for a year.

Eighty-three percent of the children were still in the study after 3 months. Over one-third of the children exhibited about 90 percent decrease in seizures. By year-end, slightly more than half of the subjects were left on the diet, and a quarter of them showed a 90 percent decrease in seizures. The research results signpost the positive effects of keto diet on children suffering from seizures. Hence, the researchers concluded that keto diets are more effective than medications in treating seizure in many instances.

It is recommended that parents should discuss the inclusion of keto diets in the menu of their children suffering from seizures with relevant medical practitioners for necessary medical advice before taking action.

KETO DIET AND BLOOD PRESSURE

One-third of American adults have been reported to experience high blood pressure. It is a serious medical problem that can cause heart attacks and strokes as increased blood pressure increases the chances of heart attacks and stroke. Adulthood and obesity increase blood pressure sensitivity.

Different medications often control high blood pressure, which sometimes has side effects on the body system. 120/80 is the best blood pressure. Although the reasons are not always clear, hypertension results in high blood pressure. The number of people suffering from high blood pressure has been on the rise due to the intensifying pressures we are facing in our lives.

It has been established that many people who suffer from high blood pressure are often recognized with excess belly fats, which increases their chances of developing type 2 diabetes. It may require a change in lifestyle to identify the fundamentals of blood pressure.

The consumption of excess carbohydrates over what the body requires can cause the symptoms of high blood pressure. This is because the consumption of carbohydrates increases the level of body sugar, and that forces the body to stimulate extra insulin, which stores fats. The excess fats lead to obesity, which can further lead to blood pressure. The intake of foods with low carbohydrates helps in reducing the blood sugar and insulin level in the body system. This basic dietary modification has a significant impact on blood pressure.

It has also been proven that potassium is of great importance when considering lowering the risk of hypertension. Medical practitioners have recommended that individuals willing to lower their blood pressure should take-in at least 4,700 milligrams of potassium daily.

Foods high in potassium are:

- Avocado
- Acorn squash
- Bananas
- Coconut water
- Dried apricots
- Pomegranate
- Salmon
- Spinach
- Sweet potato

- White beans

Although the above food items are recommended on a ketogenic diet, however, the consumption of sweet potato and beans should be moderated, due to the high carbs levels they contain.

WHAT DO I EAT ON A KETO DIET?

The keto diet is generally misconceived as it is incorrectly associated with excess fat. However, this has been proved to be the wrong stance. In keto diets, fat is converted into energy sources rather than compounding it in the body system. It is very important for us to adequately supply healthy fats to our body system that are needed for it to thrive, while other foods may not be healthier. Ketogenic diets are essential for filling the body with relevant nutrients. It is crucial to enlist the food items needed in a ketogenic diet.

As discussed earlier, the removal of processed foods and foods with high sugar content is very essential in living a healthy life. Processed foods contain preservatives that can be toxic to the human system without any benefits to offer. Hence, the reason fresh foods are highly recommended. It is also advisable that labels should be carefully read when buying new items as they can be highly informative.

Ensure carbohydrates contents in foods are not more than 50 grams daily for healthy living. A strict ketogenic diet will contain approximately 20 grams of carbs daily.

FOOD TO EAT ON A KETOGENIC DIET

- **Seafood**

Despite common knowledge of the rich content of fatty acids, vitamins, and minerals in seafood, it is not consumed by many individuals. Keto diets promote the intake of seafood. Shrimps and crabs are considered to be carb-free, while carbs are small in other shellfish.

Due to the appropriate proportion of omega-fatty acids in salmon, it is highly recommended to use sardines and other fatty fish. Fish are also known as brain food, so it is always recommended to take two or more seafood a week on a keto diet. Also recognized as seafood are simple canned tunas.

- **Vegetables**

One might wonder if a diet that promotes high leafy vegetable consumption is safe. The answer is YES because vegetables are very rich in vitamins, antioxidants, and fibers despite their low carbohydrate levels. Such rich contents make it necessary and nutritious for a healthy life. Green vegetables such as broccoli, spinach, and kale have also been shown to help reduce heart disease and cancer susceptibility. Cauliflower and turnips can also be processed to give rice-like taste and can also taste like mashed potatoes. "Starchy" vegetables, such as potatoes or beets do have carbs and should be limited on the keto diet.

- **Dairy Foods**
  - Cheeses have different tastes, and they can suit varieties of human taste. They are rich in fat content, which is necessary for energy, high in protein and calcium, and low in carbohydrates.
  - Yogurt and cottage cheese are also very rich in protein and calcium. They are low-carb, hence, a perfect fit for the ketogenic lifestyle. Ensure you only consume plain yogurt, as the low-fat versions of yogurt and the flavored types have a high content of sugar. Rather than buying flavored yogurts, one can add berries and nuts to the yogurt and cottage cheese.

- **Avocados**

Because of their rich content, avocados are also very important for a complete ketogenic diet. They have very large vitamin and mineral content, coupled with the right amount of potassium. A research study revealed that avocados are very helpful in lowering cholesterol by 22 percent. Despite its rich nutrient content and good flavor, avocados have only 2 grams of net carbohydrates. Salads and sandwiches should be added to them.

- **Meat and Poultry**

The keto diet promotes adequate quantities of meat consumption. Meat has small carbs while it is very rich in protein, enhancing the build-up of muscles. It is recommended that you always choose healthy grass-fed meats with higher fatty acids.

- **Eggs**

As they are high in protein and contain a mere 1 gram of carbohydrates, eggs are also essential for healthy living. Apart from their wealth of nutrients, they are affordable and ideal for a ketogenic diet for every individual.

Eggs are more filling, which helps to reduce the intake of food. Many have misconceptions about eating yolk, leaving them to eat just the albumen; meanwhile, the yolk is more nutritious. Hence, it is encouraged that eggs should be eaten totally.

- **Coconut Oil**

Many people are not aware of coconut oil's great importance and rich content. It is very beneficial for people with diabetes and has been used in patients with Alzheimer's disease.

In most dishes, coconut oil can also be used as a substitute for butter or oil. You can also use it for frying and sautéing.

- **Dark Chocolate**

The richness of antioxidants is an interesting fact about dark chocolate, making it one of the superfoods recommended for healthy living. In lowering blood pressure, chocolate containing more than 80 percent of real cocoa powder has been proven to be effective.

Only 10 grams of carbohydrates can be found in an ounce of 80 percent dark chocolate, making it a healthy snack to be recognized. It is important to note that for it to be classified as healthy, the proportion of cocoa content must be relatively higher. The higher the content of cocoa, the healthier the chocolate is. It is instructive to also note that milk chocolates are not classified as healthy.

FOODS TO AVOID ON A KETOGENIC DIET

One is limited to very few foods when on a keto diet, unlike other diets. Foods limited in keto diets are more likely to have high sugar content, which is why they should be avoided. This does not necessarily translate into total denial of sweet foods, there are healthy yet sweet (desserts) recipes that can be enjoyed on a keto diet. While they are to be used in small doses, some keto-friendly products such as stevia can be supplemented with traditional sweeteners in baked foods.

Also note that due to the high sugar content in them, fruit should be taken with moderation, preferably a few slices per day will be enough. Many fruit juices, though with nutrients, also have high sugar content, and concentrates that lack fiber. Therefore, reading through the fruit juice labels is important to ensure that one purchase of juices with adequate nutrients is made. It is recommended to take green juices as they are considered the best due to their low flavoring content.

One should also be mindful of cereals when on a keto diet since they are mostly packed with sugar and lack relevant nutrients. Although some of them may be marked as healthy, sugar and deficient nutrients are in a good number of them. While bran cereals are perfect for keto diets, berries can also sweeten them. It should also be noted that honey is not allowed in large quantities, and because of their sugar content, they should be limited.

White starches such as pasta, white bread, and rice, are to be exempted from one's diet as they are empty calories. However, wholegrain version can be consumed in moderation in place of white starches. While beans and legumes are healthy for the body system, they should be taken seldom due to their high carbohydrate contents (20 – 50 carb-gram a day)

Certain spirits are recommended, while some, such as alcohol, should be avoided due to their empty calories. Also, beers with high contents of carbs should be removed from the keto diet; meanwhile, wine can be taken instead. Note that wines should be checked as they vary in terms of sugar contents, dry wines have relatively small sugar contents compared to sweet dessert wines.

While Whiskey, vodka, and other pure alcohol have calories in them, they are carb-free; hence, they should be selected carefully. Also, mixing fancy cocktails with alcohols can give rise to high sugar levels; thus, they should be avoided. On the keto diet, wine coolers should not be taken as they have very high content of sugar soda with alcohol.

BOOST YOUR METABOLISM

1. Don't Overdo Calorie Cutting

Having yourself on a low-calorie diet is a surefire way of not missing out. "Your body is designed to protect your normal weight," says Liz Applegate, Ph.D., University of California professor of nutrition at Davis and founder of Bounce Its Body Beautiful. "So if you suddenly drop 1,000 calories off your diet, your resting metabolic rate [the number of calories your body burns to maintain basic body functions like breathing and heartbeat] will automatically slow down, because your body now assumes you're starving." So how many calories should you consume? Depending on your activity level, if you multiply your present weight by 11, you can safely lose from half a pound to two pounds a week, says Applegate. (For example, if you're 120 pounds, aim at around 1,320 calories a day.) Unless you're less than 5 feet tall, don't let your calories dip below 1,200 a day. "Evidence shows that women who eat less than this level find their metabolic resting rate plummeting by as much as 45 percent," reports Dale Huff, R.D., a nutritionist from St. Louis.

2. Eat Breakfast

Believe it or not, as regards metabolism (and weight loss) this may be the most important meal of the day. Breakfast eaters, according to the reports, lose more weight than breakfast skippers did. "Your metabolism slows while you're sleeping, and it doesn't come back until you're eating again," explains Barbara Rolls, Ph.D., nutrition professor at Penn State University and author of The Volumetrics Weight-Control Plan. So if you miss the meal, your body will not consume as many calories as it could until lunchtime. That's why beginning the day with a good 300-to 400-calorie meal is smart; it will jump-start your metabolism.

Look for a snack with plenty of high-fiber carbs: As researchers at the University of Sydney in Australia measured the effects of high-fat and high-fiber-carbohydrate breakfasts, they discovered that people who consumed the fatty meal got hungry earlier afterwards. "High-fiber carbs take longer for your body to digest and consume than fats; therefore, they do not induce rapid changes in your blood sugar, and the appetite is kept at bay for longer," says study co-author Susanna Holt, Ph.D. Some good choices: a bran-rich breakfast cereal with low-fat milk; whole-grain toast covered with low-fat ricotta and sliced bananas or berries; an egg-white veggie omelet with whom.

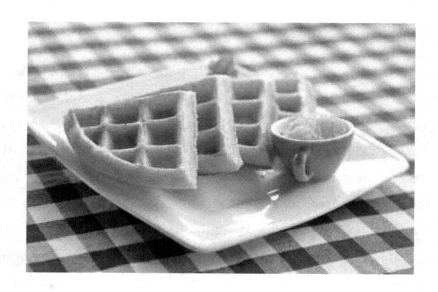

3. Pile On the Protein

Research shows you can improve your appetite by consuming plenty of protein, allowing you to lose additional 150 to 200 calories a day, says Jeff Hampl, Ph.D., R.D., a spokeswoman for the American Dietetic Association. "Protein consists mainly of amino acids, which are more difficult for your body to break down[than fat and carbs], so that you burn more calories and get rid of them," he says.

That doesn't mean you're going to have to live on the high-protein diet Atkins. Yet make sure 10 to 35 per cent of your total daily calories are protein-based. So if you're on a 1,800-calorie diet, 360 to 630 of those calories will come from lean protein products, including pork, meat, low-fat milk, yogurt and legumes. "Want to have a protein serving at every meal and snack, like nuts, a small can of tuna or a piece of low-fat string cheese," says Hampl.

4. Nibble All Day

It sounds counterintuitive; if you wanted to lose weight why would you eat continuously? But eating five to six mini meals every day, rather than three larger meals, keeps your metabolism moaning around the clock. "It'll also prevent you from going so long without food that you'll become so hungry you're overeat," Peeke says. Try not to let meals elapse for more than four hours, and make sure that each meal includes protein for an extra metabolic boost. For example, if you're eating a high-fiber cereal and fruit breakfast first, have a mid-morning snack, such as yogurt and fruit; lunch (try four ounces of chicken or fish on top of a leafy green salad); another late afternoon snack, such as a banana and a piece of low-fat cheese; and a light dinner (think four to six ounces of turkey, salmon, or another lean source of protein with steamed veggies).

5. Go for Good Carbs

Refined carbs such as bagels, white bread and potatoes create an insulin surge which in turn promotes fat storage and may drive down your metabolic rate, says Louis Aronne, M.D., an obesity specialist at the New York Presbyterian Weill Cornell Medical Center, who instead recommends high-fiber carbs. "Maintaining carbohydrates in your overall diet is significant, but focusing on vegetables, fruits and whole grains, which have less effect on insulin levels," he notes.

6. Skip Alcohol

Thinking about having a drink before dinner— or two? Talk it over again. Having a drink before a meal allows about 200 calories for people to eat, some studies show. Drinking with dinner is not such a good idea either: Other research has found that the body first burns off food, which means the calories are more likely to be processed as fat in the rest of the meal. If you have a beverage addiction, stick to alcohol that only contains a bottle of 80 calories— or reduce calories by consuming a spritzer of white wine (two ounces of wine combined with two ounces of seltzer).

7. Drink Milk

Load up on low-fat dairy: In a study published in the January 2003 American Society for Nutritional Sciences Journal of Nutrition, women who consumed milk, yogurt, and cheese three to four times a day lost 70 percent more body fat than women who did not eat milk. The reason: Calcium, along with other dairy ingredients, effectively revamps your metabolism, allowing the body to burn excess fat quicker, according to study author Michael Zemel, Ph.D., director of the University of Tennessee Nutrition Institute in Knoxville. And no, they were reinforced o.j. They're not going to do the trick. Instead of other calcium-rich foods (like broccoli), calcium-fortified products (like orange juice) or supplements, the best results come from dairy produce. Women enjoy the biggest fat-burning advantage by eating three dairy servings and 1,200 milligrams of calcium a day, Zemel's research shows.

8. Spice Up Your Soup

Sprinkle some hot peppers into your soup for lunch or stir-fry for the dinner. According to research done at the University of Laval in Canada, they temporarily boost your resting metabolic rate. Here's why: Capsaicin, a compound found in jalapeño and cayenne peppers, temporarily stimulates your body to release more stress hormones, such as adrenaline, speed up your metabolism and thus increase your ability to burn calories, says study co-author Angelo Tremblay, director of the Laval Institute of Nutraceuticals and Functional Foods. Bonus: There was less appetite for the pepper-eaters, Tremblay found, probably because the spiciness of the food made them feel full.

9. Pump Iron

Experts say weight training is the best way for your metabolic rate of rest to crank up. "When you get older, your resting metabolic rate drops, but weight training can rev it again: a pound of muscle burns up to nine times the calories a pound of fat does," fitness expert Westcott explains. In reality, a woman who weights 130 pounds and is athletic consumes more calories than a woman of the same height, sedentary to 120 pounds. Regular strength exercise will increase the metabolic rate of resting from 6.8 to 7.8 per cent everywhere. (That means you will lose about 100 extra calories a day if you weigh 120 pounds, even if you're just watching TV.) Don't you think you've got the time to hit the gym circuit? Only two 15-minute training sessions a week can deliver great results. Westcott's research, published in the January 1999 journal Medicine & Science in Sports & Exercise, found that doing only one set of 10 reps reaped the same muscle-building benefits as three sets, as long as they were performed to muscle tiredness. Bonus: Weight training also provides a short-term boost to your metabolism. As women lift weights, their metabolisms continue in overdrive after the last bench press for up to two hours, enabling them to eat as many as 100 extra calories.

10.   Rev Up Your Workouts

The introduction of strength exercise— bursts of high-intensity exercises— is a perfect fitness booster to your workout. "Studies have shown that people who do strength exercise twice a week[apart from aerobic] lose twice as much weight as those who do a daily cardio workout," says Aronne, an obesity researcher. Inserting a 30-second sprint into your jog every five minutes or adding a one-minute incline walk to your treadmill workout can easily incorporate interval training into your workout. "It's a more intense workout since your body is working harder— and so you're burning more calories," says Westcott. On other days, take 40 minutes of cross-training to shake up your routine. Ideally, plan for two interval training sessions of 20-to-40 minutes, and two cross-training sessions of 20-to-40 minutes a week.

11. Break Up Your Exercise Routine

Slice each of the exercises into 2 smaller sessions whenever possible. Do a morning weight-lifting session of 15 minutes for starters, then do a 30-minute stroll on your lunch hour or at night. That day, you'll be burning an extra 100 to 200 calories, explains Kelly Tracy, M.A., the Duke University Diet and Fitness Center fitness coordinator. Don't have enough time? Just add in some climbing stairs or short walks all day long. Even small activity bursts are enough to revive your metabolism, according to a study published in the scientific journal Nature. "I name it the mini stoke: Wake up and do something for five minutes out of every hour, even if it's just wandering around the desk," says medicine professor Peeke. "A few hundred extra calories will end up burning.

12. Sweat Out Your PMS

According to a recent study at the University of Adelaide in Australia, it is easy to curl up on the couch the minute PMS mood swings and bloat hit, but you'll lose more weight if you workout during those two weeks before your time. "For the two weeks following ovulation, people consumed approximately 30 per cent more fat than just two days before menstruating," says research coauthor Leanne Redman. Here's why: estrogen and

progesterone reproductive hormones are then at their peak —
and because they promote the body's use of fat as energy, more
fat is burned off when you exercise during this time.

13. Get Some Shut-Eye

Skimping on your sleep will ruin your metabolism. People who
got four hours of sleep or less a night had more difficulty
processing carbohydrates in a test at the University of Chicago.
"When you're exhausted, your body lacks the energy to perform
its normal day-to-day functions, including burning calories, so
your metabolism automatically decreases," Peeke explains.

According to the National Sleep Foundation, there are easy ways
to get some good night's sleep. Have your exercises planned early
in the day; exercise within two to three hours of bedtime will
keep you asleep. And try to soak in a hot bath, since studies show
that warm water makes sleeping easier.

14. Chill Out

Long-term stress can make you fat, research has found. "The
body gets filled with stress hormones when you're excessively
stressed, which cause fat cells deep in the belly to increase in size
and promote fat storage," Peeke says. "I call this toxic weight

because fat is more likely to increase your risk of heart disease, diabetes and cancer deep inside your belly." And stress hormones spark your appetite, making you more likely to over-consume.

What to do, then, is a frazzled woman? Make a list of all the things that relax: play with the puppy, write in your journal, even listen to classical music. Then encourage yourself to sit back and enjoy one of those things for 10 to 15 minutes each day.

15. Treat Yourself

When you cut calories to lose weight, add 200-300 to your daily intake every once in a while, says Amanda Bonfiglio Cunningham, a senior teacher in yoga medicine. "The body will get used to a calorie-deficit diet, adjusting by slowing down the metabolic rate. You're creating a healthy balance by allowing yourself a day of indulgence (not overindulgence!), she explains. "The extra calories elevate the production of leptin, a hormone that regulates appetite and energy. This elevation triggers thermogenesis, the natural tendency of the body to create heat that results in calories being burned."

16. Go Green (Tea)

Until you chuck somebody's head over a French press, read on. You don't have to quit caffeine — but add in the mix a pair of cups of green tea and you may think your trousers match a little looser. "Research shows the potential of caffeine and catechin in green tea to increase the metabolic rate by 4-5 percent and boost fat oxidation by 10-16 percent," Bonfiglio Cunningham says. Green tea comes with an additional benefit, too — its antioxidant properties. "The antioxidants present in many teas battle free radicals in the body, improve the process of ageing and reduce the risk of disease."

17. Joke Around

Take the funny cat videos-according to experts, they're good for your health. Unfortunately, you're not going to get the same calorie-burning effects as you get from your spin class, but laughing does give a small boost to your metabolism. A study published in the International Journal of Obesity found that genuine laughter increased energy expenditure and heart rate above resting values by 10-20 per cent. Another study has found that especially watching cat videos can boost your energy level. Guess you know from now on what you are watching on the treadmill.

18. Drink Water — and Lots of It

It might seem so convenient to improve your metabolism by drinking water but it really does. Researchers found in a study published in The Journal of Clinical Endocrinology and Metabolism the metabolisms of participants improved by just 10 minutes after consuming 16 ounces of H20 by a whopping 30 per cent.

19. Try a Low-Glycemic Diet

Consider a diet rich in vegetables, grains, and legumes instead of eating carbohydrates or going low-fat to improve your metabolism— to prevent the blood sugar from spiking. "Most people think that weight is all about calories in, calories out, but also about consistency," says Aunna Pourang, M.D. In a 2012 study] low-carb diets showed the biggest rise in metabolism but also elevated stress hormone cortisol, which is why scientists concluded that the low-glycemic diet worked best."

20.   Add Healthy Fats to Your Meals

Eating fats may sound scary when you're trying to speed up your metabolism — but you just have to eat the right type. To see a shift focus on a balanced diet of protein, grains, and healthy fats such as avocados, almonds, and olive oil.

GETTING STARTED ON THE KETO DIET

It's very easy and seamless to start a keto diet. As one would be exposed to amazing health benefits, embracing a keto diet is a very commendable thought and decision with the numerous benefits attached to the diet. Here's the stuff you need to kick-start a keto diet.

- **Clear Your Pantry**

The first thing is to clear your sight of sugar and carbs. Although one might be strongly willing and so determined to stay away from carbs and sugar, the reality is that one will be tempted to return to sugar intake if one looks at them frequently. You should clear up your kitchen to avoid temptations after you decide to go on a keto diet. You can also humbly ask your family to limit the intake of sugar and carbs in the house so as not to discourage you.

- **Weigh Yourself**

It is also recommended to track the weight of the body. Sometimes, because of additional healthy body muscles, you may feel like you're adding weight. This is why it is recommended that you, perhaps once a week, check your weight to monitor your progress.

- **What About Your Favorite Meals?**

It might feel scared that you are giving up your favorite meal for a keto diet. Meanwhile, keto diet will not deprive you of your favorite meal; every meal has a perfect substitute, which has low carbs content. Even mashed potatoes and cheesecake have their relevant substitute that gives the same taste despite their low carbs content.

Most food items that are labeled low fats or low carbohydrates can be deceiving. In fact, labels can be deceiving no matter the degree of attention we pay when reading product labels. Sometimes, it requires a level of expertise before one can fully understand them. Sugars are added to the acclaimed low fat and low carbohydrates food in most stores; hence, it is advised that one should avoid such products completely.

- **Always Stay Hydrated**

As the kidney excretes more liquid during a keto diet, it is also essential to take enough water to stay hydrated, hence the need for adequate water intake. The low level of insulin causes the excretion of liquid.

- **Condiments Can Be the Enemy**

Condiments such as ketchup, salad dressings, and more should also be avoided due to the high level of sugar in them. It is important to read labels and avoid low-fat versions because their sugar contents are higher.

It is safe to go with salad dressing to your restaurant when planning to take salad in an eatery. You can also ask the attendants about the ingredients of their salad dressing to ensure you avoid high sugar intake.

- **Keep Track of Your Ketone Level**

Tracking how the body responds to keto diets is very essential. One can do a simple urine test, and a blood ketone meter can be purchased. The test is best performed in the morning.

- **Friends and Family Can Be Annoying – Bless Their Hearts**

Sometimes, family members and friends may not understand the keto diets; they may also consistently insist that you try something sweet or with high sugar content. You don't need to put up fights against them, take some avocados, nuts, and other ketogenic foods instead. Also, you should remain firm with your decision and stick to your diet.

It will take resolve to stick to your diet. It may help to fill up on keto-friendly snacks before you sit down and eat. Enjoy some nuts, an avocado, or just a leg of chicken before you eat, and you will be less tempted.

- **Celebration**

At times, one might be stuck in a tricky situation, especially celebration moments such as birthdays, anniversary, and even surprises from colleagues or family members. In cases like this, it can really be a dicey one as it will be difficult to turn people down.

Here is a tip of how one can handle that. Express your greatest excitement at that moment and let them feel the appreciation of their kind gesture. Afterward, look for an excuse to move from the center of the activity, you can declare your desire to have a coffee. Most likely, people will be too carried away to notice that you have not taken out of the cake.

- **Traveling**

When on a keto diet, getting healthy foods while traveling may not come that easy. Hence, it is necessary to take a few things such as a blender, bananas, avocados, and other low carbs items with you. Some tuna and anchovies can also be taken.

- **Eating Out**

When eating out, you can consider sticking to meat, vegetables, while avoiding noodles and potatoes. In a Chinese restaurant, you can always opt for egg foo young, steamed fish with vegetables, clear soups, among others. You can also request that the attendants should exclude cornstarch from your meal.

You can eat the meat in your burger alone if the eatery does not have a salad. You can also try it when in a friend's house.

- **Exercise**

A keto diet helps with muscle mass building, in addition to the supply of body energy. Thus, it is advised that one should include exercises, such as walking more, joining a gym class, or taking the stairs in daily routines.

TIPS AND GUIDELINES

The ultimate goal of a ketogenic diet is to get the body into a certain metabolic state known as ketosis. As mentioned earlier, when your body depletes all the glycogen stores, it turns to the fat stores to produce ketones that in turn give the cells in your body energy. It suggests that the energy source for your body is no longer the carbohydrates but the ketones.

But there seems to be an issue here—many people who begin the ketogenic diet have a difficulty reaching the ketosis state or remaining in ketosis state after they get in! We also force themselves out of that state of ketosis. If you avoid the mistakes Amateurs make, you can overcome this.

Common mistakes to avoid

- **Don't be scared of fat**

If you want to shed your extra fat then you need to get fatter. Sounds stupid? Well, not if you heard that-" You've got to spend money to make money!" Keto follows a similar logic-to get into ketosis, the body needs more dietary fat and considerably fewer dietary carbohydrates. If you want to transform the body into a fat-burning engine, then you should rid it of carbohydrates first (primary source of energy: glycogen–retained glucose). When you do that, your body feels it hasn't been getting enough glucose through food and so begins to use the glucose (glycogen) that has been stored. Once it exhausts the reserve completely, it starts looking for a new source of energy.

The body approaches the accumulated body fat and splits the fatty acids down into it. These fatty acids form ketones. When this happens, your body is going into a completely new metabolic state–ketosis! In reality eating good fats will help you get rid of all the water weight and excess flab. So you could eat butter and cheese.

- **Water is important**

To keep your body hydrated you need to regularly drink enough water throughout the day. The medical experts conventional recommendation is–you need to drink at least one gallon of water each day to support the body's organ function properly and do its respective job!

It may be tough if you are a busy worker but my advice to you is to keep a glass of clean drinking water next to your office. Hold on sipping it as often as you can. If you have water near you, you tend to drink more water of course than you usually do!

You may need to visit the restroom frequently but that's fine, as your body will get used to your new drinking routine over a period of time and handle things accordingly.

- **Get Salty**

If you're a keto dieter for the first time you could feel some of the effects of keto flu. Constant headaches, fatigue, feeling feverish, etc. −but you don't need to worry, because your body is trying to adapt to a new routine, you get these symptoms. Those flu-like symptoms can definitely be prevented!

As you eat real, wholesome food and drink loads of water, you lose more electrolytes. No junk things and artificial preservatives get into your body. There's some cleansing activity going on in your body−so you have to help your body by replenishing the lost electrolytes.

How are you? The best way to achieve this is to add salt (sodium) to your blood. You should blend the drinking water with a teaspoon of salt, and have it once a day. As they have salt, you should add sriracha or chili garlic sauce to your diet too. You should apply a little bit of salt while giving your salads or other dishes extra seasoning.

There's another advantage of drinking more salt−the body can retain water easily, thereby reducing your bathroom trips.

- **Dairy is good but don't go overboard**

The ketogenic diet protocol is to include a large amount of high-fat food items and the most commonly used source of high-fat food is—full-fat dairy.

The dilemma here is, when you drink too much milk (more than the necessary amount of calories), you immediately begin to realize that you've reached a plateau. You are not losing any more weight at this point. Why? For what? The theory here is-if you need to lose weight, you need to put your body in a calorie deficit mode, i.e. you need to give it less calories.

For example—if your body burns around 1500 calories per day and you consume 1000 calories per day, your body needs to find the remaining 500 calories to burn now. You give that to your body in the form of fat, when you're in keto. Returning to our dairy products—since most dairy items are calorie-rich, over-eating is quite natural for you, resulting in calorie overload. That means—you don't allow your body to use the extra fat for more nutrition, as you already fuel it with the food you need.

It is good to add a good amount of mozzarella to your meals but don't eat the whole mozzarella block in one go.

- **Know your WHY factor**

The important part of any diet is-you ought to know why you do it. Do you have a specific diet, because you want to look good? Or do you do it to improve the overall health? Whichever cause you need to fix it in your mind is good. Your psychology accounts for 99 percent of your dietary success-your mental capacity should be strong! You need to be exactly why you do it, and believe it's going to succeed!

You may often get tempted to eat stuff that drives you out of ketosis. During those times you have to think about your WHY. Your goal, your goal is key! When you steal once it's cool, don't fret over it. Think positive-ask yourself the question, why am I not expected to get back on track? I can get back on board and soon arrive at my destination.

The WHY should inspire you to reach your goal, and move you ahead. It has a genuinely strong emotion.

- **Too much protein isn't good**

This is another reason the body goes out of the state of ketosis. Since meat can be included in your diet, there are times when you tend to over-eat the meat dishes. Through gluconeogenesis process too much protein may produce glucose. The body first converts to glycogen excess protein and converts the glycogen into fat.

It's good to add chicken breast to your daily regimen, but eating a whole bucket of chicken fry actually won't do any good for your keto diet. To stop these situations remember to take care of your regular macros. If not, buy less meat while you go shopping for your grocery.

- **Stop snacking often**

Too much snacking will knock you out of ketosis, because your blood sugar levels can spike up. The good thing about a keto diet is that you include a decent amount of high fat in your meals and you feel satiated. Therefore, particularly when you have added more fiber to your food platter, the urge to get snacks that.

A handful of energy almonds is good but not a bowl of cashews! The best way to reduce too much snacking is to prepare your meal well in advance of your meal so you don't indulge in snacking while cooking your meal.

- **No more habit-eating**

One of the best things about keto diet is getting better control over your appetite. Many people in need of something to eat listen to their stomach growl and walk towards the fridge or pantry. To avoid giving in to your cravings you should give up that habit. After 2 to 3 weeks on keto diet you may not feel these items.

But there may be few people experiencing a hiccup here—since you have been eating in a particular way for some time, you get used to that habit. You might be used to eating something after every three hours, for example, and this habit of eating will now take you to the fridge even if you're not hungry. You need to work actively to turn your mind off to that habit. By planning your meals much earlier, the best way to achieve this is-meal plan plays an important role in the keto diet.

- **Sleep is essential**

If you don't give the much-needed rest to your mind and body, your system will face trouble doing things that it is supposed to do. Good quality sleep is important for controlling your stress, giving your organs rest and making you feel energetic the next day.

Eight hours of sleep is compulsory and, thankfully, a well-planned keto diet will give you the sleep you require without any problems. But just don't blame me if you're a party animal.

- **Stress management**

To over-stress yourself will increase the levels of cortisol in your body. What exactly is cortisol? The stress hormone increases the level of your blood sugar which hinders your weight loss plan.

It sends a confusing signal to your brain when your body experiences a successive rise and fall in blood sugar levels.

Naturally, your brain assumes it's time to refill the glycogen reserve and so it sends you a signal saying it needs carbs now! When it's under stress, your body craves sugar. This is that body's survival mechanism! If you want a successful keto journey then work on your stress management needs to be done.

- **Don't eat the same meal every time**

You have to mix up your recipes or you'll get hungry too easily. There are so many keto-friendly recipes out there and you just have to choose the ones that are best for you. You can also discover your own new recipes by adding gastronomic expertise to your touch. To your regular keto dinner, add some low-carb vegetables and season them with herbs and condiments.

Why would you want to have the same lunch and dinner for the whole month when there are numerous options available? Unleash your imagination, and make your kitchen a laboratory of innovation.

- **No cheat days**

There are few diets that offer you cheat days so that on that one day you can wolf down all your favorite things. But be patient-in keto there are no easy days. This is a strict dietary regimen and if you want to maintain your goal weight you have to stick to its guidelines. If you feel like a sponge cake or chocolate with milk, make a fat bomb, and have it.

Keto offers you an almost all-substitute. Be aware of your errors, and prepare accordingly. Planning your meals is key to preventing these commonly repeated errors. It's not that easy to get out of it once you get into ketosis so remaining on it is not easy either.

KEY PILLARS GOING FORWARD

- **Water**

Water has no calories, fat, or cholesterol and has low levels of sodium. It is nature's appetite suppressant, and it helps the body to metabolize fat, thereby helping you lose weight.

- **Fiber**

There is a slew of health benefits that come with consuming lots of dietary fiber. They include: normalizing bowel movements and maintaining bowel health, lower blood cholesterol levels, helps control blood sugar levels, promote healthier gut bacteria and reduce risk of certain cancers

- **Rest and Sleep**

Going forward, adequate rest and sleep will become a major pillar in your quest to lead a healthy lifestyle. The importance of sleep and rest cannot be overstated. Among its numerous benefits include: Appetite regulation, reducing your calorie intake, increases your resting metabolism, prevents insulin resistance and provide you with energy for physical activity

- **Positive Mindset**

A positive mindset can help you maintain your plant-based diet and realize your health and fitness goals. Seeing as this requires patience and commitment, having a positive outlook and approach is going to help you: stay motivated, focus on the positive aspects of your diet, and overcome emotions during your low moments.

- **Physical Activity**

The health benefits of regular exercise and physical activity are hard to ignore. Exercising regularly will help you: Control weight fights off health conditions and diseases, improve your mood, boost your energy levels and promote better sleep

BREAKFAST AND BRUNCH CHAFFLES RECIPES

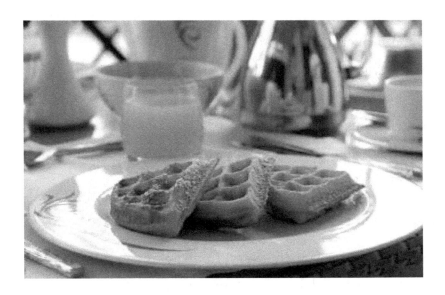

1. Italian cream chaffle cake recipe

This recipe makes about 8 mini waffles, or you can use a big waffle maker and it will make 3 to 4 waffles! If you don't want to do a big batch, feel free to cut the recipe in half.

Sweet Chaffle Ingredients

- 4 oz Cream Cheese, softened and room temp
- 4 eggs

- 1 tablespoon melted butter
- 1 teaspoon vanilla extract
- ½ teaspoon cinnamon
- 1 tablespoon monkfruit sweetener (or your favorite keto-approved sweetener)
- 4 tablespoons coconut flour
- 1 tablespoon almond flour
- 1 ½ teaspoons baking powder
- 1 tablespoon coconut, shredded and unsweetened
- 1 tablespoon walnuts, chopped

Italian Cream Frosting Ingredients:

- 2 ounces cream cheese, softened and room temp
- 2 tablespoons butter, room temp
- 2 tablespoons monkfruit sweetener (or your favorite keto-approved sweetener)
- ½ teaspoon vanilla

Preparation

- Add the cream cheese, eggs, melted butter, vanilla, sweetener, coconut flour, almond flour, and baking powder in a medium-sized blender. Optional: add or save the melted coconut and walnuts to the mixture for the frosting.

- Mix the ingredients till it is rich and smooth.
- Mini-waffle machine preheat.
- Apply the preheated ingredients to the waffle maker.
- Cook before the waffles are done, for around 2 to 3 minutes.
- Replace the chaffles and let them cool off.
- Continue preparing the frosting in a different bowl by putting all ingredients together. Stir until moist and smooth.
- Frost the cake until the chaffles are fully cool.
- Serve.

2. Keto taco chaffle ingredients (makes 2 chaffles)

Ingredients

- ½ cup cheese (cheddar or mozzarella), shredded
- 1 egg
- 1/4 teaspoon Italian seasoning

Taco meat seasonings for 1 lbs of ground beef

- 1 teaspoon chili powder
- 1 teaspoon ground cumin
- ½ teaspoon garlic powder
- ½ teaspoon cocoa powder
- ¼ teaspoon onion powder
- ¼ teaspoon salt
- 1/12 teaspoon smoked paprika

Preparation

- First, cook the ground beef or turkey.
- Stir in all seasonings of taco meat. The cocoa powder is optional but the tastes of all other seasonings are completely improved!

- Continue preparing the keto chaffles while you are cooking the taco rice.
- Waffle machine to preheat.
- First shake the egg in a tiny bowl.
- Cover with shredded cheese and seasoning.
- Put half the mixture into the mini waffle maker and cook for 3 to 4 minutes.
- Save and prepare the second half of the paste in order to make a second chop.
- Apply the moist taco meat to the saucepan.
- Cook your ground beef or turkey first with the lettuce, tomatoes, cheese and serve warm
- First, boil your ground beef or turkey.
- Stir in all seasonings of taco meat. The cocoa powder is optional but the tastes of all other seasonings are completely improved!
- Continue preparing the keto chaffles while you are cooking the taco meat.
- Waffle machine to preheat.
- First shake the egg in a tiny bowl.
- Top with shredded cheese and seasoning.
- Put half the mixture into the mini waffle maker and cook for 3 to 4 minutes.

- Save and prepare the second half of the paste in order to make a second chop.
- Add the warm taco meat to the saucepan.
- Complete with salad, onions, cheese and serve warm

3. Easy chicken parmesan chaffle

Chaffle Ingredients

- ½ cup canned chicken breast or leftover shredded chicken
- ¼ cup cheddar cheese
- 1/8 cup parmesan cheese
- 1 egg
- 1 teaspoon Italian seasoning
- 1/8 teaspoon garlic powder
- 1 teaspoon cream cheese, room temperature
- Topping Ingredients:
- 2 slices of provolone cheese
- 1 tablespoon sugar-free pizza sauce

Preparation

- Mini-waffle machine preheat.
- Put all the ingredients in a medium-sized pot, and blend until fully incorporated.
- Fill the waffle iron with a teaspoon of shredded cheese for 30 seconds before adding the mixture.
- This will create the best crust and make it easier for the waffle maker to pull it strong chaffle out when it's finished.

- Pour half of the mixture into the mini waffle maker and cook for 4 to 5 minutes or more.
- Follow the steps above for cooking the second Parmesan Chicken Chaffle.
- Complete with 1 slice of provolone cheese and a sugar-free pizza sauce. With even more Italian Seasoning I like to dust the rim too.

4. Cheesy garlic bread chaffle recipe ingredients (makes 2 cheesy garlic bread chaffles)

Garlic Bread Chaffle Ingredients

- ½ cup mozzarella cheese, shredded
- 1 egg
- 1 tablespoon Italian seasoning
- ½ tablespoon garlic powder
- 1 tablespoon cream cheese

Garlic Butter Topping Ingredients

- 1 tablespoon butter
- ½ tablespoon Italian seasoning
- ½ tablespoon garlic powder
- Cheesy Bread Topping
- 2 tablespoon mozzarella cheese, shredded
- Dash of parsley (or more Italian seasoning)

Preparation

- Have your mini waffle maker preheated.
- Preheat the oven until 350F.
- Mix all the garlic bread chaffle ingredients together in a small bowl until well blended.
- Split the mixture into two, and cook the first mixture for at least 4 minutes. If you like chopping on the outside a bit

crunchy, it's advisable to put a tablespoon of shredded cheese on the waffle maker for 30 seconds before adding the ingredients to the chaffle. This will create a beautiful, crunchy crust that is pretty stunning.

- The garlic bread chaffles in the waffle maker are moved to a baking sheet after you cook them out.
- Melt the butter over the microwave for about 10 seconds in a separate small bowl.
- Stir in the butter mixture with the garlic butter seasonings.
- Apply the butter mixture with a basting brush over moist chaffles.
- Sprinkle on the garlic bread chaffles a small amount of mozzarella and sprinkle with more Italian seasoning.
- Bake to 350F degrees for 5 minutes. This is just enough time to melt the cheese on top of Chaffles Cheesy Garlic Bread.
- Serve warm and savor with a sugar-free marinara sauce like Rao's Marinara sauce.

5. Chickfila copycat chaffle sandwich

Ingredients for the chicken:

- 1 Chicken Breast
- 4 tablespoons of Dill Pickle Juice
- 2 tablespoons Parmesan Cheese, powdered
- 2 tablespoons Pork Rinds, ground
- 1 tablespoons Flaxseed, ground
- Salt and Pepper
- 2 tablespoons Butter, melted

Ingredients for chaffle sandwich bun:

- 1 Egg (room temperature)
- 1 cup Mozzarella Cheese, shredded
- 3 -5 drops of Stevia Glycerite
- ¼ teaspoon Butter Extract

Preparation

Instructions for the chicken

- Chicken pound to ½ centimeter thick.
- Cut in half and put baggie with pickle juice in a zip lock.

- Close the baggie and placed in the refrigerator for 1 hour to overnight.
- Preheat Air-fryer for 5 minutes at 400
- Blend the Parmesan cheese, pork rinds, flaxseed and S&P together in a tight, shallow bowl.
- Cut the chicken and remove the pickle juice from the baggie.
- Sprinkle the chicken in a melted butter mixture and then season.
- Put parchment paper round in Airfryer tub; lightly brush the paper with oil. (I used coconut)• Put chicken in Airfryer preheated and cook for 7 minutes.
- Flip the chicken and Airfry for another 7-8 minutes. (This may vary depending on your chicken size) 165 Internal Tempo

Instructions for chaffle bun:

- Mix everything in a small bowl. Place ¼ of the mixture into the waffle iron with preheated mini tap. Cook 4 mins. Move to a rack to cook. Repeat x3
- Assemble Sandwich's: place the resting chicken on one Chaffle bun, add 3 slices of dill pickle. Certain buns render. Replicate. Love it!

6. Keto cornbread chaffle

Ingredients

- 1 egg
- ½ cup cheddar cheese, shredded (or mozzarella)
- 5 slices jalapeno, optional – picked or fresh
- 1 teaspoon frank's red hot sauce
- ¼ teaspoon corn extract (this is the secret ingredient that is a must!)
- Pinch salt

Preparation

- Mini waffle machine preheat
- Heat the egg in a small bowl.
- Add the remaining ingredients and combine until well-integrated.
- Fill the waffle maker with a tablespoon of shredded cheese for 30 seconds before adding the mixture. That will make an absolutely fantastic fresh and crisp crust!
- Add half of the mixture to preheated waffle manufacturer.
- Bake for at least 3 to 4 minutes. The longer you cook it, the more it gets crispy.
- Serve warm, and have fun.

7. Keto chaffle stuffing recipe ingredients (makes 4 chaffles)

Basic Chaffle ingredients

- ½ cup cheese, mozzarella, cheddar or a combo of both
- 2 eggs
- ¼ tablespoon garlic powder
- ½ tablespoon onion powder
- ½ tablespoon dried poultry seasoning
- ¼ tablespoon salt
- ¼ tablespoon pepper

Stuffing ingredients

- 1 small onion, diced
- 2 celery stalks
- 4 oz mushrooms, diced
- 4 tablespoon butter (for sauteing)
- 3 eggs

Preparation

- Make the chaffles, first. This dish is made with 4 mini chaffles.
- Preheat iron with mini waffle.
- Preheat the oven to 350F

- Mix the diced vegetables in a medium-size dish.
- Pour ¼ of the mixture into a mini waffle maker, and cook for about four minutes each.
- Lay them aside once they're all cooked.
- Saute the cabbage, celery, and mushrooms in a small frying pan until they are tender.
- Tear the chaffles into small pieces in a separate bowl, and then add the sauteed veggies and 3 eggs. Mix until the components are thoroughly come together.
- Add the stuffing mixture to a small saucepan (about 4x 4) and bake at 350 degrees for 30 to 40 minutes or so.
- Serve warm, and have fun

8. **Keto birthday cake chaffle recipe (makes mini four cakes)**

Chaffle Cake Ingredients:

- 2 eggs
- ¼ cup almond flour
- 1 teaspoon coconut flour
- 2 tablespoons melted butter
- 2 tablespoons cream cheese, room temp
- 1 teaspoon cake batter extract
- ½ teaspoon vanilla extract
- ½ teaspoon baking powder
- 2 tablespoons swerve (confectioners sweetener or monkfruit)
- ¼ teaspoon Xanthan powder

Whipped Cream Vanilla Frosting Ingredients:

- ½ cup heavy whipping cream
- 2 tablespoons swerve (confectioners sweetener or monkfruit)
- ½ teaspoon vanilla extract

Preparation

- Mini-waffle machine preheat.
- Put all the chaffle cake ingredients in a medium-sized blender and mix on high until it is smooth and creamy. Let the batter rest just for a minute. It may seem a little watery but it's just going to work perfectly.
- Add 2 to 3 teaspoons of flour to your waffle maker and cook until it is golden brown for around 2 to 3 minutes.
- Continue making the whipped vanilla frosting cream in a separate bowl.
- Add all the ingredients and mix together with a hand mixer until the whipping cream is thick and soft peaks form.
- Allow chaffles from the keto birthday cake to cool completely before frosting your cake. When you ice it out too soon, the frosting will melt.
- Enjoy!

9. Keto sausage ball chaffle recipe

Ingredients

- 1 pound bulk Italian sausage (no need to precook the sausage either)
- 1 cup almond flour
- 2 teaspoons baking powder
- 1 cup sharp cheddar cheese, shredded
- ¼ cup Parmesan cheese, grated
- 1 Egg or if you have an egg allergy you can use the Flax Egg technique (1 T ground flax seed mixed with 3T of water)

Preparation

- Mini-waffle machine preheat.
- Pour all ingredients into a large mixing bowl and use your hands to combine properly.
- Put a sheet of paper under the waffle maker to contain any spillage.
- On hot waffle maker, scoop 3 T of mixture.
- Cook, for at least 3 minutes. Flip over, and cook for even crispiness for 2 more minutes.

10.   Banana nut chaffle recipe

Ingredients

- 1 egg
- 1 tablespoon cream cheese. softened and room temp
- 1 tablespoon sugar free cheesecake pudding (optional ingredient because it is dirty keto)
- ½ cup mozzarella cheese
- 1 tablespoon Monkfruit confectioners
- ¼ tablespoon vanilla extract
- ¼ tablespoon banana extract

Optional Toppings:

- Sugar free caramel sauce
- Pecans (or any of your favorite nuts)

Preparation

- Mini waffle machine preheat
- Heat the egg in a small bowl.
- Add the remaining ingredients to the egg mixture and mix until well embedded.
- Add half of the batter to the waffle maker, and cook for at least 4 minutes until golden brown.

- Remove the finished mixture and add the other half of the mixer to cook the other mash.
- Complete with the ingredients of your choosing and serve warm!
- Enjoy!

11. Pumpkin cake chaffle

Ingredients

- 1 egg
- ½ cup mozzarella cheese
- ½ tablespoon pumpkin pie spice
- 1 tablespoon pumpkin (solid packed with no sugar added)
- Optional Cream Cheese Frosting Ingredients:
- 2 tablespoon cream cheese, softened and room temperature
- 2 tablespoon monkfruit confectioners blend (or any of your favorite keto-friendly sweetener)
- ½ tablespoon clear vanilla extract

Preparation

- Preheat the mini-waffle maker.
- Heat the egg in a small saucepan.
- Add ham, pie seasoning and pumpkin spice.
- Mix in well.
- Apply ½ of the mixture to the mini waffle maker and cook for 3 to 4 minutes or more until golden brown.
- In a cup, add all the cream cheese frosting ingredients and mix until it is smooth and creamy, when cooking. You can

also add a tablespoon of real butter that has been softened at room temperature, if you want a buttery taste to this frosting.

- Apply the frosting cream cheese to the hot chop and serve immediately.

12.Strawberry shortcake chaffle recipe

Ingredients

- 1 egg
- ¼ cup mozzarella cheese
- 1 tablespoon cream cheese
- ¼ tablespoon baking powder
- 2 strawberries, sliced
- 1 tablespoon strawberry extract

Preparation

- Waffle machine to preheat.
- Heat the egg in a small saucepan.
- Using ingredients left over.
- Spray non-stick cooking spray into the waffle maker.
- Split the mixture into two.
- Fry half of the mixture for about 4 minutes, or until chocolate golden.

13. Pumpkin cake chaffle

Ingredients

- 1 egg
- ½ cup mozzarella cheese
- ½ tablespoon pumpkin pie spice
- 1 tablespoon pumpkin (solid packed with no sugar added)

Optional Cream Cheese Frosting Ingredients:

- 2 tablespoon cream cheese, softened and room temperature
- 2 tablespoon monkfruit confectioners blend (or any of your favorite keto-friendly sweetener)
- ½ tablespoon clear vanilla extract

Preparation

- Mini-waffle machine preheat.
- Whip the egg in a small saucepan.
- Add cheese, cake spice and pumpkin spice.
- Mix in well.
- Apply ½ of the mixture to the mini waffle maker and cook for 3 to 4 minutes or more until golden brown.

- In a bowl, add all the cream cheese frosting ingredients and mix until it is smooth and creamy, while cooking. To this frosting, if you want a buttery taste, you can also add a tablespoon of real butter which has been softened at room temperature.
- Add the frosting cream cheese to the hot chop and serve immediately.

14. Crispy everything bagel chaffle chips

Ingredients

- 3 tablespoons Parmesan Cheese or Parmigiano Reggiano, shredded
- 1 teaspoon Everything Bagel Seasoning

Preparation

- Mini-waffle machine preheat.
- Put the Parmesan cheese on the griddle and let it burst. Around 3 minutes. Make sure to leave it long enough or, when it cools, it won't turn crispy. Important move!
- Sprinkle another 1 tablespoon of melted cheese with Everything Bagel Seasoning. Leave open the waffle iron while it's frying!
- Unplug the mini-waffle maker and let it cool down for a few minutes. This will cause the cheese to cool enough to become crispy and bind together.
- It'll still be moist after only 2 minutes of it cooling off.
- Use a mini spatula to peel the moist (but not hot) waffle iron cheese.
- Allow crispy chips to cool off absolutely

15. Keto blt chaffle sandwich

Ingredients

Chaffle bread ingredients

- ½ cup mozzarella, shredded
- 1 egg
- 1 tablespoon green onion, diced
- ½ tablespoon Italian seasoning
- Sandwich ingredients
- Bacon, pre-cooked
- Lettuce
- Tomato, sliced
- 1 tablespoon mayo

Preparation

- Mini waffle maker preheat
- Whip the egg in a small bowl.
- Blend in cheese, seasonings, and onions. Mix until it's fully put in.
- In a mini waffle maker, put half the batter and cook for 4 minutes.
- If you want a crunchy sandwich, add a tablespoon of shredded cheese for 30 seconds before applying the batter

to the mini waffle iron. The extra cheese is making the perfect crust on the outside!

- Add the remaining batter to the mini waffle maker after the first chopping is complete and cook for 4 minutes.
- Top the sandwich with the mayo, ham, cabbage, and tomato.
- Enjoy!

16.Cilantro Jalapeno Dip Recipe

Ingredients

- 6 to 8 jalapenos
- 1 bushel cilantro meaning a huge handful
- 1 packet of dry Ranch dressing mix
- 1 cup Sour Cream
- 1 cup Mayonnaise

Preparation

1. Puree the jalapenos and cilantro in a food processor until it appears like a paste
2. Be sure to pick out the jalapenos seeds if you like a mild dip
3. Blend the cilantro and jalapeno puree blend together with 1 cup of mayonnaise and 1 cup of sour cream mixture
4. Wait for about an hour and eat
5. Enjoy!

Tip: Use that too on burgers! It's just great.

17. Chocolate chip cookie chaffle cake

Ingredients for cake layers:

- 1 tablespoon butter, melted
- 1 tablespoon Golden Monkfruit sweetener
- 1 egg yolk
- 1/8 teaspoon vanilla extract
- 1/8 teaspoon cake batter extract
- 3 tablespoons almond flour
- 1/8 teaspoon baking powder
- 1 tablespoon chocolate chips, sugar free

Whipped Cream Frosting Ingredients:

- 1 teaspoon unflavored gelatin
- 4 teaspoon cold water
- 1 cup heavy whipping cream
- 2 tablespoons confectioners sweetener

Preparation

Chocolate chip cookie chaffle cake

- Mix all in a mini waffle iron and cook for 4 minutes. Repeat with layer after layer. I opted to make 3.

Whipped cream frosting instructions

- Put the beaters and mixing bowl in the freezer for about 15 minutes so they can cool.
- Sprinkle the gelatin over cold water in a microwave-safe cup. Cut, and let "bloom" It takes about 5 minutes.
- The gelatin mixture microwave for 10 seconds. It becomes a liquid. Stir to ensure it's all dissolved.
- Start whipping the cream at a low speed in your cold mixing bowl. Add sugar to the confectioner's.
- Switch to a higher speed and search for strong peaks to start forming.
- At max whipping cream, turn back to lower level and gradually drizzle the molten liquid gelatin mixture in. Once it is in, switch back to a higher speed and continue to beat until stiff peaks are reached.
- Place your cake in a piping bag and pipe it.

Note: For this recycling I used only ½ of the whipped cream.

18.Keto red velvet waffle cake recipe

Ingredients

- 2 tablespoons Dutch Processed Cocoa
- 2 tablespoons Monkfruit Confectioner's
- 1 egg
- 2 drops super red food coloring (optional)
- ¼ tablespoon Baking Powder
- 1 tablespoons heavy whipping cream
- Frosting ingredients
- 2 tablespoons Monkfruit Confectioners
- 2 tablespoons Cream Cheese, softened and room temp
- ¼ tablespoon clear vanilla

Preparation

- Whip up the egg in a small bowl.
- Add the remaining ingredients and stir well until the batter is creamy and smooth.
- In a mini waffle maker, add half the batter and cook for 2½ to 3 minutes until it is fully cooked;
- Put the sweetener, cream cheese, and vanilla in a single, small bowl. Mix up the frosting until all is well integrated.
- Spread the frosting over the waffle cake after it has cooled down completely to room temperature.

19. Chicken jalapeno popper chaffle (makes 2 chaffles)

Ingredients

1. ½ cup canned chicken breast
2. ¼ cup cheddar cheese
3. 1/8 cup parmesan cheese
4. 1 egg
5. 1 small jalapeno, diced (fresh or pickled)
6. 1/8 tablespoon onion powder
7. 1/8 tablespoon garlic powder
8. 1 tablespoon cream cheese, room temperature

Preparation

1. Preheat the mini-waffle maker.
2. Put all the ingredients in a medium-sized pot, and blend until fully incorporated.
3. Pour half of the mixture into a mini waffle maker and cook for 4 to 5 minutes or more.

Additional Toppings: sour cream, hot sauce, ranch dressing, cilantro, green onion, feta cheese or jalapeno.

20. Keto boston cream pie chaffle cake recipe (makes mini four cakes)

Ingredients

Chaffle Cake Ingredients:

- 2 eggs
- ¼ cup almond flour
- 1 teaspoon coconut flour
- 2 tablespoons melted butter
- 2 tablespoons cream cheese, room temp
- 20 drops Boston Cream extract
- ½ teaspoon vanilla extract
- ½ teaspoon baking powder
- 2 tablespoons swerve (confectioners sweetener or monkfruit)
- ¼ teaspoon Xanthan powder

Custard Ingredients:

- ½ cup heavy whipping cream
- ½ teaspoon Vanilla extract
- ½ tablespoon Swerve confectioners Sweetener
- 2 Egg Yolks
- 1/8 teaspoon Xanthan Gum

Ganache Ingredients:

- 2 tablespoons heavy whipping cream
- 2 tablespoons Unsweetened Baking chocolate bar, chopped
- 1 tablespoon Swerve Confectioners Sweetener

Preparation

- Preheat mini waffle iron to first make cake chaffles.
- Mix all the ingredients of the cake in a mixer and mix in fast until it is smooth and creamy. That should only take a few minutes.
- Heat the heavy whipping cream over the stovetop to a boil. While heating, whisk together the egg yolks and Swerve in a separate tiny bowl.
- Garnish half of it in the egg yolks once the cream is boiling. Make sure you whisper together whilst slowly mixing in the mixture.
- In the leftover milk, add the egg and cream mixture back into the stovetop pan and stir vigorously for another 2-3 minutes.
- Take off the heat of the custard and sweep in the vanilla & xanthan gum. Then set it aside to freshen and thicken.

- Put ingredients in a small bowl for the ganache. Microwave, run for 20 seconds. Repeat if appropriate. Be vigilant not to overheat and roast the ganache. Do only 20 seconds at a time until it is melted to the full.
- Assemble your Chaffle Cake Boston Cream Pie and enjoy.

LUNCH AND DINNERS CHAFFLES RECIPES

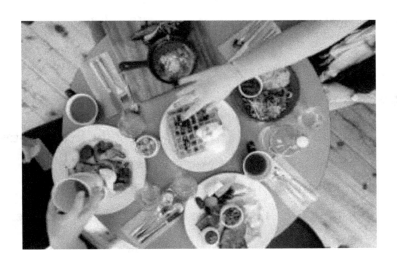

1. Corndog chaffle recipe

Ingredients

- Flax Egg – Mix 1 T ground flaxseed with 3 T water
- Set aside to rest (If you're not allergic to egg whites skip the flax and use 1 large egg)
- 1½ T Melted Butter
- 2 tablespoons sweetener, granulated
- 3 T Almond Flour
- ¼ tablespoon Baking Powder
- 1 Egg Yolk
- 2 T heaping Mexican Blend Cheese

- 1 T chopped Pickled Jalapeños
- 15 -20 drops Cornbread Flavoring
- Extra cheese for sprinkling on waffle maker

Preparation

- Mix all of that together. Let them rest for five minutes. If it is too dense, add 1 T of water, or HWC.
- Sprinkle the waffle maker with shredded cheese on the bottom. Add 1/3 of that batter. Sprinkle over with shredded cheese.
- Waffle iron locks.
- Don't press them back.
- Take off when the cheese is crisp. Replicate. Serves 3.

2. Keto pizza chaffle recipe

Ingredients

- 1 egg
- ½ cup mozzarella cheese, shredded
- Just a pinch of Italian seasoning
- No sugar added pizza sauce (about 1 tablespoon)
- Top with more shredded cheese, pepperoni (or any of your favorite toppings)

Preparation

- Dash waffle machine preheat.
- Whip the eggs and seasonings together in a small bowl.
- In a shredded cheese mixture.
- Add the preheated waffle maker with a tsp of shredded cheese and allow to cook for about 30 seconds. That will help create a crisper crust.
- Add half the mixture to the waffle maker and cook until golden brown and slightly crispy for about 4 minutes!
- Remove the waffle and add the remaining mixture to the waffle maker.
- Top with pizza sauce, shredded cheese, and pepperoni. Microwave it for about 20 seconds on fast, and voila! Fast Pizza chaffle!

3. Sloppy Joe chaffle recipe

Ingredients

- 1 lb ground beef
- 1 tablespoon of onion powder (you can substitute for 1/4 cup real onion)
- 1 tablespoon of garlic, minced
- 3 tablespoon of tomato paste
- 1/2 tablespoon of salt
- 1/4 tablespoon of pepper
- Tablespoon of chili powder
- 1 tablespoon of cocoa powder (this is optional but highly recommended! It intensifies the flavor!)
- ½ cup bone broth (beef flavor usually)
- 1 tablespoon of coconut aminos (or soy sauce if you prefer)
- 1 tablespoon of mustard powder
- 1 tablespoon of Swerve brown (or Sukrin golden)
- ½ tablespoon of paprika

Cornbread chaffle ingredients (Makes 2 chaffles)

- Egg
- ½ cup cheddar cheese
- 5 slices jalapeno, diced very small (can be pickled or fresh)
- 1 tablespoon Franks Red Hot Sauce

- ¼ tablespoon corn extract (optional but tastes like real cornbread!)
- Pinch salt

Preparation

- Cook the ground beef first with salt and pepper.
- Apply the ingredients left over.
- Allow the mixture to simmer while the chaffles are being made.
- Waffle machine to preheat.
- Whip the egg in a small saucepan.
- Use ingredients left over.
- Sprinkle nonstick cooking spray to the waffle maker.
- Divide the blend into half.
- Fry half of the mixture for about 4 minutes, or until slightly colored.
- Add 1 tablespoon of waffle cheese to the waffle maker for 30 seconds before adding the mixture for a crispy outer crust on the chaffle.
- Sprinkle the moist sloppy Joe mixture on a hot chaffle and voila! Dinner is served.

4. Keto lemon chaffle recipe

Ingredients

Chaffle Cake:

- 2 oz cream cheese, room temp and softened
- 2 eggs
- 2 tablespoon of butter, melted
- 2 tablespoon of coconut flour
- 1 tablespoon of monkfruit, powdered confectioners blend (add more if you like it sweeter)
- 1 tablespoon of baking powder
- ½ tablespoon of lemon extract
- 20 drops cake batter extract

Chaffle Frosting:

- ½ cup heavy whipping cream
- 1 tbs monkfruit, powdered confectioners blend
- ¼ tablespoon of lemon extract

Preparation (this recipe makes about 4 chaffles)

- Preheat the mini waffle maker

- Apply all the chopped cake ingredients to the blender and combine until the batter is smooth and pleasant. That should only take a few minutes.
- Use an ice cream scoop, then line the waffle iron with a full batter scoop. The ice cream scoop is about 3 teaspoons of this size and fits perfectly in the mini waffle maker.
- Start making the frosting while the chaffles are frying.
- Add the frosting ingredients for the chaffle in a medium-sized bowl.
- Mix the ingredients with peaks until the frosting is thick.
- All the chaffles are to cool completely before the cake is frosted.

Optional: Add lemon peel for additional flavour.

Chaffle Tip: Use an ice cream scoop to accurately weigh the batter out.

5. Keto peanut butter chaffle cake recipe

Ingredients

Peanut Butter Chaffle Ingredients:

- 2 tablespoons Sugar Free Peanut Butter Powder
- 2 tablespoons Monkfruit Confectioners Keto Sweetener
- 1 egg
- ¼ teaspoon Baking Powder
- 1 tablespoon Cream Cheese, softened
- ¼ teaspoon Peanut Butter extract

Peanut Butter Frosting ingredients

- 2 tablespoons Monkfruit Confectioners Keto Sweetener
- 1 tablespoon Butter, softened and room temp
- 1 tablespoon sugar free natural peanut butter or peanut butter powder
- 2 tablespoons Cream Cheese, softened and room temp
- ¼ teaspoon vanilla

Preparation

- Whip up the egg in a small bowl.

- Add the remaining ingredients and stir well until the batter is thick and smooth.
- You can skip this if you don't have the peanut butter extract. It adds a more intense flavor to peanut butter that is absolutely wonderful and makes the extract worth investing in.
- Pour half the batter into a mini waffle maker and cook for 2 to 3 minutes until it's cooked completely.
- Put the sweetener, cream cheese, sugar-free natural peanut butter and vanilla into a separate small pot. Mix up the frosting until all is well integrated.
- Spoon the frosting over the waffle cake after it has cooled down entirely to room temperature.
- Or pipe the frosting too!
- Or you can heat the frosting and apply a ½ tablespoon of water to make it a peanut butter glaze that you can cut over your peanut butter chaffle too!

6. Oreo cookie chaffle recipe

Ingredients

Chaffle ingredients:

- 1 egg
- 1 tablespoon black cocoa powder
- 1 tablespoon monkfruit confectioners blend (or your favorite keto-approved sweetener)
- ¼ teaspoon baking powder
- 2 tablespoons cream cheese, room temperature and softened
- 1 tablespoon mayonnaise
- ¼ teaspoon instant coffee powder (not liquid)
- Pinch salt
- 1 teaspoon vanilla

Frosting ingredients:

- 2 tablespoons monkfruit confectioners
- 2 tablespoons cream cheese softened and room temp
- ¼ teaspoon vanilla

Preparation (this recipe makes 3 OREO chaffles)

- Whip up the egg in a small bowl.

- Add the remaining ingredients and stir well until the batter is creamy and smooth.
- Divide the batter into 3 and pour each into a mini waffle maker and cook until fully cooked for 2½ to 3 minutes.
- Add the sweetener, cream cheese, and vanilla in a separate, small bowl. Mix up the frosting until all is well integrated.
- Spoon the frosting over the waffle cake after it has cooled down entirely to room temperature.

7. Keto chaffle recipe

Ingredients

- ½ c. shredded cheese
- Pinch of salt
- Seasoning to taste
- large egg

Preparation

- Preheat the mini-waffle maker.
- Whisk the egg in a mug, until it is pounded.
- Shred the cheese (they like any flavor or combination).
- Add the egg to the milk, salt and pepper, and blend properly.
- At the waffle maker, scoop half the mixture, spread evenly.
- Cook 3-4 minutes, until cooked (crispy) to your liking.
- Remove, and let it cool.
- Pour in the remaining batter and cook the 2nd waffle. Enjoy!

8. Keto chaffle churro recipe

Ingredients

- 1 egg
- ½ cup mozzarella cheese, shredded
- 2 tablespoons Swerve Brown Sweetener
- ½ teaspoon cinnamon

Preparation

- Preheat iron with mini waffle.
- Heat the egg in a tiny bowl with a fork.
- Add the egg mixture to shredded cheese.
- Put half the egg mixture in the mini waffle maker and cook until it is golden brown (about 4 minutes)
- Apply the Swerve Brown Sweetener and cinnamon in a separate small bowl while the mini Chaffle is frying.
- Once the Chaffle has been done, cut it into slices (as shown in the video) while it is still hot and add it to the mixture of cinnamon. When it is still hot it soaks up more of the mixture!
- Serve warm and enjoy!

9. Keto chocolate waffle cake recipe

Ingredients

- 2 tablespoon of Cocoa
- 2 tablespoon of Monkfruit Confectioner's
- 1 egg
- ¼ tablespoon of Baking Powder
- 1 tablespoon of heavy whipping cream

Frosting ingredients

- 2 tablespoons of Monkfruit Confectioners
- 2 tablespoons of Cream Cheese, softened and room temp
- ¼ tablespoon of clear vanilla

Preparation

- Whip up the egg in a small bowl.
- Add the remaining ingredients and stir well until the batter is creamy and smooth.
- In a mini waffle maker, add half the batter and cook for 2 1/2 to 3 minutes until it is fully cooked;
- Put the sweetener, cream cheese, and vanilla in a single, small bowl. Mix up the frosting until all is well blended.

- Spoon the frosting over the waffle cake after it has cooled down entirely to room temperature.

10.   Keto vanilla twinkie copycat chaffle recipe

Ingredients

- 2 tablespoons butter, melted (cooled)
- 2 ounces cream cheese, softened
- 2 large eggs (room temp)
- 1 teaspoon vanilla extract
- 1/2 teaspoon Vanilla Cupcake Extract (optional)
- 1/4 cup Lakanto Confectioners
- Pinch of pink salt
- 1/4 cup almond flour
- 2 tablespoons coconut flour
- 1 teaspoon baking powder

Preparation

- Preheat the Corndog Maker.
- Melt butter for a minute, and let it cool.
- In oil, whisk the eggs until creamy;
- Mix in coffee, sugar, sweetener, salt and blend well.
- Add almond flour, baking powder and coconut flour.
- Mix until well put in.
- Add 2 tablespoons of batter to each well and spread evenly across it.

- Close the lid, lock and let it cook for four minutes.
- Remove from the rack and cool off.

11. Buffalo chicken chaffle recipe

Ingredients

- 1 Can Valley Fresh Organic Canned Chicken Breast (5 ounces)
- 2 T Red Hot Wing Sauce
- 2 oz Cream Cheese, softened
- 4 T Cheddar Cheese, shredded
- 2 T Almond Flour
- T Nutritional Yeast
- ½ tablespoon of Baking Powder
- 1 Egg Yolk (Can Use whole egg if no allergy)
- 1 Flax Egg (1 T ground flaxseed, 3 T water)
- ¼-½ Cup Extra Cheese for the waffle iron

Preparation

- Process the egg flax and set aside to rest.
- Pour out the canned chicken milk. Blend all the ingredients. Sprinkle over the waffle iron with a little bacon. Let it set for a few seconds before adding 3 T of mixture to chicken. (I used a large cookie scoop) Then add a little more cheese to the waffle iron before closing. Cook for five minutes.

- Don't open the waffle iron before the time is up or you're going to get messy. Remove and let cool until hot sauce drizzle and ranch dressing is applied.

12. Keto smores chaffle recipe

Ingredients

For the Chaffles (makes 2 slices):

- 1 large Egg
- ½ c. Mozzarella cheese, shredded
- ½ tablespoon Vanilla extract
- 2 tablespoons Swerve, brown
- ½ tablespoons Psyllium Husk Powder (optional)
- ¼ tablespoons Baking Powder
- Pinch of pink salt
- ¼ Lily's Original Dark Chocolate Bar
- 2 tablespoons Keto Marshmallow Creme Fluff Recipe

Preparation

- Make the Keto Marshmallow Creme Fluff batch
- Whisk the egg until it is creamy.
- Mix in coffee and Swerve Red, and blend properly.
- Mix and stir in the shredded cheese.
- Next apply Psyllium husk concentrate, salt and baking powder.
- Mix and let the batter rest for 3-4 minutes until well incorporated.

- Prep / plug in to preheat your waffle maker.
- Apply ½ batter to the waffle maker and cook for 3-4 minutes.
- Lift and attach to a rack for cooling.
- Cook the same batter for the second half, then remove to cool.
- Assemble the chaffles until cold with a marshmallow fluff and candy:
- Using 2 tbs of marshmallow and ¼ bar of chocolate lily.
- Eat as is, or melty toast and gooey Smore sandwich!

13. Jicama hash brown chaffle recipe

Ingredients

- 1 large jicama root
- ½ medium onion, minced
- 2 garlic cloves, pressed
- 1 cup cheese of choice (I used Halloumi)
- 2 eggs, whisked
- Salt and Pepper

Preparation

- Peel jicama • Shred in food processor
- In a broad colander put shredded jicama, sprinkle with 1-2 tablespoon of salt. Mix well, and let drain.
- Squeeze out as much liquid as possible (very important step)
- Microwave for 5-8 minutes
- Combine all ingredients together
- Sprinkle some cheese on waffle iron before applying 3 T of the mixture, sprinkle a little more cheese on top of the mixture
- Cook for 5 minutes. Flip and add 2 more to prepare.
- Finish the egg with a sunny side up

14. Low carb waffle bowl recipe

Ingredients

- 1 egg. whipped
- 1 scoop Ketologic Meal, Chocolate
- 1 tablespoon almond flour
- ¼ teaspoon baking powder

Preparation

- • Preheat and spray the Bowl Waffle Maker with nonstick cooking spray.
- In a small bowl, shred the egg. Whip away the egg.
- Add the Ketologic Meal, almond meal and baking powder.
- Blend until the components are completely come together.
- Place the ingredients around a minute to a minute and a half in the preheated bowl waffle maker. Once you see the steam emerges from the pump, you'll know it's nearly done.
- Using tongs to cut the Maker's hot waffle pot.
- Let it cool and have fun.

15. Krispy kreme copycat chaffle recipe

Ingredients

Krispy Kreme Copycat Donut Chaffle Ingredients

- 1 egg
- ¼ cup mozzarella cheese, shredded
- 2 T cream cheese, softened
- 1 T sweetener
- 1 T almond flour
- ½ tablespoon Baking Powder
- 20 drops glazed donut flavoring by OOOFlavors
- Raspberry Jelly Filling Ingredients
- 1/4 cup raspberries
- 1 tablespoon chia seeds
- 1 tablespoon confectioners sweetener

Donut Glaze Ingredients

- 1 tablespoon powdered sweetener
- A few drops of water or heavy whipping cream

Preparation

Make the chaffles:

- Put everything together first to make the chaffles.

- Cook for 2 1/2-3 minutes approx.

Make the Raspberry Jelly Filling:

- Blend over medium heat in a small pot.
- Mash the raspberries, gently.
- Let them cool down.
- Remove both Chaffle boards.

Make the Donut Glaze:

- Mix in a small dish.
- Chaffle Drizzle on top.

16. Carrot chaffle cake recipe

Ingredients

Carrot Chaffle Cake ingredients

- ½ cup carrot, shredded
- 1 egg
- 2 T butter, melted
- 2 T heavy whipping cream
- 3/4 cup almond flour
- 1 T walnuts, chopped
- 2 T powdered sweetener
- 2 tablespoons of cinnamon
- 1 tablespoon pumpkin spice
- 1 tablespoon baking powder

Cream Cheese Frosting

- 4 oz cream cheese, softened
- ¼ cup powdered sweetener
- 1 tablespoon vanilla extract
- 1-2 T heavy whipping cream (depending on the consistency you prefer)

Preparation

- Mix your dry ingredients, including almond flour, cinnamon, pumpkin spice, baking powder, powdered sweetener and pieces of walnut.
- Add carrot, egg, melted butter, heavy cream to the wet ingredients.
- Add 3 T batter to Mini Waffle Maker. Cook 2 minutes ½-3.
- Combine the frosting ingredients with a hand mixer and whisk attachment until well combined.
- Line the waffles and apply every coat of frosting.

17. Banana pudding chaffle cake

Ingredients

Pudding Ingredients

- 1 large egg yolk
- ½ cup heavy whipping cream
- 3 T powdered sweetener
- ¼ – ½ tablespoon xanthan gum
- ½ tablespoon banana extract

Banana Chaffle Ingredients

- 1 oz cream cheese, softened
- ¼ cup mozzarella cheese, shredded
- 1 egg, beaten
- 1 tablespoon banana extract
- 2 T sweetener
- 1 tablespoon baking powder
- 4 T almond flour

Preparation

- In a small saucepan, add the heavy cream, powdered sweetener and egg yolk.

- Continuously whisk until sweetener dissolves and the mixture thickens.
- 1 minute soak.
- Add the whisk and xanthan gum.
- Remove from heat and stir well with a pinch of salt and the banana extract.
- Transfer to a glass platter and cover the pudding surface with plastic wrap.
- To cool.
- Mix ingredients.
- Cook in mini waffle maker, preheated.

18.Cap'n crunch cereal chaffle cake recipe

Ingredients

- 1 egg
- 2 tablespoons almond flour
- ½ teaspoon coconut flour
- 1 tablespoon butter, melted
- 1 tablespoon cream cheese, room temp
- 20 drops Captain Cereal flavoring
- ¼ teaspoon vanilla extract
- ¼ teaspoon baking powder
- 1 tablespoon confectioners sweetener
- 1/8 teaspoon xanthan gum

Preparation

- Preheat the mini-waffle maker.
- Mix all the ingredients together until smooth and creamy. Allow the batter to rest in the flour for a few minutes to absorb the liquid.
- Add 2 to 3 spoonful of batter to your waffle maker and cook for 2½ minutes.
- Top with fresh whipped cream (I added 10 drops of flavored Captain cereal) and syrup

19.Jicama loaded baked potato chaffle recipe

Ingredients

- 1 large jicama root
- 1/2 medium onion, minced
- 2 garlic cloves, pressed
- 1 cup cheese of choice
- 2 eggs, whisked
- Salt and Pepper

Preparation

- Strip jicama and shred in food processor
- In a broad colander put shredded jicama, sprinkle with 1-2 tsp of salt. Mix well, and let drain.
- Squeeze out as much liquid as possible (very important step)
- Microwave for 5-8 minutes
- Mix all ingredients together
- Sprinkle some cheese on waffle iron before adding 3 T of the mixture, sprinkle a little more cheese on top of the mixture
- Cook for 5 minutes. Flip and add 2 more to prepare.
- Top with a dollop of sour cream, pieces of bacon, cheese and chives.

20.   Fried pickle chaffle sticks recipe

Ingredients

- 1 egg, large
- ¼ cup pork panko
- ½ cup mozzarella
- 1 tablespoon pickle juice
- 6-8 thin pickle slices

Preparation

- Mix in the mix.
- Add waffle iron to a thin layer.
- Blot excess pickle juice.
- Add the pickle slices and then add another thin mixing layer.
- Cook for 4 minutes.

BASIC FLAVORED CHAFFLES RECIPES

1. Buffalo Cauliflower Bites

Ingredients

Blue cheese dressing

- 1/3 cup of sour cream
- 1 tablespoon of avocado oil mayonnaise
- ¼ teaspoon of coarse salt
- ¼ teaspoon of garlic powder
- 2 tablespoons of crumbled blue cheese

Buffalo sauce

- 2 tablespoons of unsalted butter
- ¼ cup of hot sauce
- ½ teaspoon of garlic powder

Buffalo cauliflower

- 1 lb. fresh of cauliflower florets
- 2 tablespoons of olive oil
- ½ teaspoon of coarse kosher salt (not fine salt)
- ½ teaspoon of garlic powder

Preparation

- Heat the oven to 450 degrees F. Line a parchment paper to a rimmed broiler-safe baking sheet.
- Blue cheese dressing: in a small bowl, combine all the ingredients. Cover and cool.
- Buffalo sauce: melt the butter. Whisk in the powdered garlic and hot sauce. Set aside.
- Cauliflower: Put the cauliflower with the olive oil, salt and garlic powder in a large bowl. Spread on the baking sheet and roast until tender-crisp (15 min.) Switch the oven to broil and place a 6-inch oven rack under the heat element.
- Whip the hot sauce mixture. Add the florets of the roasted cauliflower and coat. Return the cauliflower to the baking sheet and cook until bubbly browned, 2-3 minutes.

2. Keto Zucchini Boats

Ingredients

- 4 medium Zucchini
- 2 tablespoon of Olive oil
- Sea salt
- 1/3 cup diced Onion
- 1 lb minced pork sausage
- 2 cloves Garlic
- 14.5 oz Diced tomatoes
- 1/3 cup Grated Parmesan cheese
- 1 tablespoon of Italian seasoning
- 1 cup shredded Mozzarella cheese

Preparation

- Heat the oven to 400F/200C. Line a foil or parchment paper on a baking sheet.
- Slice the courgettes longitudinally. Use a spoon to cut some of the zucchini's centers.
- Put on the baking sheet. Drizzle with a spoon of olive oil and sprinkle with sea salt. Roast for approximately 15-20 minutes in the oven until soft.
- In a large non-stick skillet, steam 1 tablespoon of olive oil over medium-high heat. Add the onions that have been diced. Saute until brown for about 10 minutes. Add the

pork sausage and cook until browned for about 10 minutes. Attach the chopped garlic and saute for a minute or so. Remove the sausage from heat. Add onions, grated Parmesan, and Italian seasoning. Put in the zucchini boats with the sausage mixture. Sprinkle with shredded mozzarella.

- Bake until the cheese is melted, this should be between 5-10 minutes.

3. Keto raspberry cheesecake brownies

Ingredients

- 4 oz. unsweetened baking chocolate, chopped
- 6 oz. butter
- 1 cup erythritol
- 4 large eggs
- 1 cup almond flour
- 2 tablespoons of vanilla extract
- ¼ tablespoon of salt
- 10 oz. cream cheese, softened
- 1/3 cup powdered erythritol
- 1 large egg
- 2 tablespoons of vanilla extract
- 1 tablespoon of raspberry extract (optional)
- 1 tablespoon of lemon juice
- 6 oz. fresh raspberries

Preparation

- The oven should be heated to 350 ° F/175 ° C. Line a parchment-paper to a baking dish.
- On a low heat melt the chocolate and butter. Stir in the sweetener.

- Combine eggs, almond meal, vanilla extract and salt in a large bowl. Remove the melted mixture of chocolate and whisk together. In the ready pot, pour the mixture.
- Mix cream cheese and powdered sweetener with a mixer until soft and smooth. Add in the egg and blend well. Add the vanilla extract, raspberry extract and lemon juice and fold in the fresh raspberries gently. Drop large spoonful of the cheesecake mixture over the brownie batter. Swirl the cheesecake batter horizontally and vertically into the brownie batter.
- Bake for 35-40 minutes or until set.

4. Low-Carb Bacon and Cheese Egg Muffins

Ingredients

- 6 eggs
- Salt and pepper to taste
- 6 slices of Butcher Box bacon, cooked
- 1/4 cup onion, chopped
- 1/4 medium green pepper, chopped
- 1/4 medium red pepper, chopped
- 1/4 cup shredded mozzarella cheese
- 1/4 cup shredded cheddar cheese
- 1/4 cup fresh spinach, finely chopped

Ingredients

- Heat the oven to 350 degrees.
- In a large bowl, whisk the eggs with salt and pepper. Spray cooking oil on a 12-capacity muffin tin. Pour the eggs (about halfway) into each tin.
- The bacon, onions and peppers can be mixed in a bowl. Place the vegetables on the eggs. Top with shredded cheese.
- Bake until the eggs are ready this should take about 14-16 minutes.

5. Keto cauliflower soup with crispy pancetta

Ingredients

- 4 cups chicken broth or vegetable stock
- 1 lb cauliflower
- 7 oz. Cream cheese
- 1 tablespoon of dijon mustard
- 4 oz. Butter
- Salt and pepper
- 7 oz. Pancetta or bacon, diced
- 1 tablespoon of butter, for frying
- 1 tablespoon of paprika powder or smoked chili powder
- 3 oz. Pecans

Preparation

- Cut the cauliflower into smaller florets. The smaller you slice them, the quicker it gets ready for the broth.
- Save tiny 1/4 inch pieces of fresh cauliflower and chop them into bits.
- Cook the fine-cut cauliflower (from step 2) and pancetta or bacon until crispy. Towards the end, add nuts and paprika powder. Set the mixture aside to serve.
- Cook the cauliflower in the stock until tender. Add butter, mustard and cream cheese.

- Blend the soup to the desired consistency with the immersion blender. The longer you mix the soup, the more creamy the soup. Add salt and pepper to taste.
- Serve the soup in bowls and cover with the fried pancetta mixture.

6. Keto harvest pumpkin and sausage soup

Ingredients

- 1½ lbs fresh sausage
- 1/3 cup minced red onions
- 1/3 cup diced red bell peppers
- 1 minced garlic clove
- 1 pinch salt
- ½ tablespoon of rubbed dried sage
- ½ tablespoon of ground dried thyme
- ½ tablespoon of red chili peppers flakes (optional)
- ½ cup pumpkin puree
- 2 cups chicken broth
- ½ cup heavy whipping cream
- 2 tablespoons of salted butter

Preparation

- On medium-high heat, use a large skillet to brown the bacon, onion and pepper.
- Sprinkle in the seasonings and stir to blend when pork is thoroughly cooked and onions and pepper are brown (about 10 to 15 minutes).
- Pour in the milk, broth and pumpkin. Let is simmer uncovered for 15 to 20 minutes at low heat or until the broth is thickened.

- Stir well in butter and serve warm.

7. Keto no-noodle chicken soup

Ingredients

- 4 oz. butter
- 2 tablespoon of dried minced onion
- 2 celery stalks, chopped
- 6 oz. mushrooms, sliced
- 2 minced garlic cloves
- 8 cups chicken broth
- 1 medium sized carrot, sliced
- 2 tablespoons of dried parsley
- 1 tablespoon of salt
- ¼ tablespoon of ground black pepper
- 1½ rotisserie chicken, shredded
- 5 oz. green cabbage, sliced into strips

Preparation

- Melt the butter over medium-heat in a large pot.
- In the pot, add dried onion, celery, sliced mushrooms and garlic and cook for 3-4 minutes.
- Add carrot, parsley, salt and pepper to the broth. Let it simmer until the vegetables are tender.
- Add cooked chicken and cabbage. Simmer for another 8-12 minutes until the cabbage "noodles" are soft.

8. Low-carb Goulash soup

Ingredients

- 1 yellow onion
- 2 garlic cloves
- 8 oz. celery root or rutabaga
- 1 red bell pepper
- 1 lb ground lamb or ground beef
- 4 oz. butter or olive oil
- 1 tablespoon of paprika powder
- ¼ tablespoon of cayenne pepper
- 1 tablespoon of dried oregano
- ½ tablespoon of crushed caraway seeds
- 1 tablespoon of salt
- ¼ tablespoon of ground black pepper
- 14 oz. crushed tomatoes
- 2½ - 3 cups water
- 1½ tablespoon of red wine vinegar

For serving

- 1 cup sour cream or mayonnaise
- Fresh parsley, for garnish

Preparation

- Peel and finely chop the vegetables.
- Fry the onion and garlic in a pan over medium heat with a generous quantity of oil or butter until softened.
- Add the ground meat and sauté until cooked and browned, stirring occasionally.
- Add bell pepper, paprika, celery root, cayenne, oregano, caraway, salt and pepper. Stir for approximately 1 minute. Pour in the tomatoes and 2 cups of water.
- Raise heat and gently boil the broth. Let it cook for 10 minutes.
- Before serving, add the remaining water and vinegar.
- Serve with sour cream or mayonnaise dollop and finely chopped parsley.

9. Creamy low-carb broccoli and leek soup

Ingredients

- 1 leek
- 2/3 lb broccoli
- 2 cups water
- 1 vegetable bouillon cube
- 7 oz. Cream cheese
- 1 cup heavy whipping cream
- ½ tablespoon of ground black pepper
- ½ cup fresh basil
- 1 garlic clove, pressed
- Salt

Cheese chips

- 4½ oz. cheddar cheese or edam cheese
- ½ tablespoon of paprika powder

Preparation

Broccoli soup

- Thoroughly rinse the leek and chop the green and white parts finely. Cut off the broccoli's core and slice thinly. Divide and reserve the remaining broccoli into smaller florets.

- In a pan filled with water, put the leek and sliced broccoli core. Add the bouillon cube. Season with salt and bring to a boil over high heat for a few minutes until a knife pierces the broccoli stem easily.
- Add the broccoli florets. Lower the heat and cook until the broccoli is bright green and tender for a few minutes. Add cream cheese, salt, pepper, basil and garlic.
- Mix to the desired consistency with the immersion blender.
- If the soup is too thick, add water to the broth. If you want the consistency to be slightly thicker, add a touch of heavy cream.

Cheese chips

- Fit a big, parchment-paper onto a rimmed baking sheet. Grate the cheese and put the mounds with a table spoon on the parchment. Leave 1 inch between the mounds of cheese.
- Top each cheese mound with paprika.
- Bake in the oven for about 5-6 minutes at 400 ° F (200 ° C) until the cheese has melted. Enjoy with a snack or a soup.

10. KETO avocado boats

Ingredients

- 2 avocados halved with pit removed
- 4 medium eggs
- 2 strips of bacon diced and cooked till crispy
- Salt and pepper to taste
- Chopped fresh herbs for garnish

Preparation

- Preheat the oven up to 400 F.
- Line a baking sheet. To create a larger nest for the eggs, slice avocados in half and scoop an extra 1-2 tablespoons of avocado flesh.
- Place the avocado halves on the baking dish. Carefully break an egg in each half of the avocado.
- Bake until the whites are set and the egg yolks cooked to your taste this should be about 13-18 minutes. Garnish with herbs (optional) and cover the egg cups with some crispy bacon.

11. Gazpacho Soup

Ingredients

- 6 cups chopped tomatoes (4–5 medium tomatoes)
- 2 cups chopped peeled cucumber
- 1 cup chopped red onion (1/4 red onion)
- 1/3 cup chopped fresh parsley
- 1/3 cup chopped fresh basil
- 2 tablespoons lemon juice
- 1 tablespoon of extra-virgin olive oil
- 1 teaspoon of salt
- 1/4 teaspoon of black pepper
- 1/2 cup grape tomatoes, quartered

Preparation

- In a food processor or high powered blender, add the 6 cups of tomatoes, 1 ½ cup cucumber, 3/4 cup red onion, ¼ cup parsley, ¼ cup basil, lemon juice, olive oil, salt and pepper and process until liquefied.
- Then add in remaining chopped vegetables and chill for 1 hour before serving.
- Garnish with remaining herbs. Enjoy!

12. Keto basil pesto

Ingredients

- 2 cups Fresh Basil Pressed into measuring cup
- 4 Garlic Cloves
- 1/3 cup pine nuts
- 2/3 cup grated parmesan cheese
- 1/2 cup olive oil
- 1 teaspoon of Salt
- 1 teaspoon of Pepper

Preparation

- Put the basil, garlic, pine nuts, and parmesan cheese into a food processor. Pulse until chunky. Add the Olive oil in slowly whilst the food processor is still on, until it has all been added.
- Add the salt and pepper. Enjoy!

13. Keto Teriyaki Chicken

Ingredients

- 2 Tablespoons Avocado oil
- 2 1/2 Pounds Chicken thighs cut into pieces
- 1/4 Cup Soy sauce
- 3 Tablespoons Brown sugar substitute
- 1 Clove garlic, minced
- 1 teaspoon Grated ginger
- 1/2 Cup water
- 1/4 teaspoon Xanthan gum
- Sesame seeds, sliced green onions and red pepper - optional/garnish

Preparation

- Heat the avocado oil in a large skillet over medium heat. Add the chicken and sauté' until cooked through for about 8 minutes.
- In a bowl combine the soy sauce, sugar substitute, garlic, ginger, water, and xanthan gum. Whisk to combine. Pour the sauce into the skillet with the chicken and reduce the heat to medium. Continue cooking for a few more minutes until the sauce thickens and coats the chicken.
- Serve topped with sesame seeds, sliced green onions and pepper for garnish. Enjoy!

14. Keto Double Chocolate Muffins

Ingredients

- 2 cups almond flour
- 3/4 cup unsweetened cocoa powder
- 1 1/2 tsp. baking powder
- 1/4 cup swerve sweetener
- 1 tsp. salt
- 1 cup melted butter
- 3 large eggs
- 1 tsp. pure vanilla extract
- 1 cup sugar-free dark chocolate chips

Preparation

- Heat the oven to 350 degrees.
- Put the almond flour, cocoa powder, sweetener, baking powder and salt in a pan and whisk. Add the butter, eggs and vanilla and blend until combined. Add the chocolate chips
- Bake until a toothpick inserted in the middle comes out clean this should take about 12 minutes.

15. Keto chicken quesadilla

Ingredients

- 1 1/2 Cups Mozzarella Cheese
- 1 1/2 Cups Cheddar Cheese
- 1 Cup Cooked Chicken
- 1/4 Cup Bell Pepper
- 1/4 Cup Diced Tomato

Preparation

- Preheat oven to 400 F. Cover a pan with Parchment Paper.
- Mix the Mozzarella and Cheddar cheese together. Spread them over the parchment paper. Bake the cheese shell for 5 min.
- Put more than half of the cheese shell in the chicken. Add the sliced tomato and peppers. Cut the Cheese shell in half over the chicken and veggies.
- Press firmly. Return it to the oven for 4- 5 min. Serve with sour cream, salsa and guacamole.
- Garnish with basil, parsley or coriander. Enjoy!

16. Dutch pancakes with berries

Ingredients

- 3 tablespoons almond flour
- 1 teaspoon of Swerve
- Pinch of salt
- 1 egg
- 3 tablespoons almond milk
- 1/4 teaspoon vanilla extract
- 1 teaspoon butter
- Handful of berries
- 1 tablespoons of cream cheese

Preparation

- Heat the oven to 400° F.
- In a small cast iron skillet, put the butter and melt over low heat.
- Whisk the swerve, sugar, egg, almond milk and vanilla until smooth. Pour into the skillet and transfer to the oven.
- Bake the berries and cream cheese for 10 minutes.

17. Keto zucchini noodles

Ingredients

- 4-5 medium-sized zucchini
- 1 lb/ 450 gr. Raw shrimp peeled and deveined
- 3 tablespoons of butter
- Salt and pepper to taste
- 4 garlic cloves finely chopped
- 1 lemon juice and zest
- 1 teaspoon Italian seasoning
- 1/2 teaspoon smoked paprika

Preparation

- Make the zucchini noodles.
- Heat the butter in a large pan over medium-high heat. Add the shrimp in a single layer and season with salt and pepper. Cook for about 1-2 minutes.
- Add the garlic, then flip the shrimp for another 1-2 minutes, or until pink. Then add lemon juice, Italian seasoning and paprika. Transfer the shrimp to a plate leaving the sauce in the pan.
- Add zucchini to the pan and toss for about 30 seconds to a minute.
- Add the shrimp back to the pan and toss again until everything is warmed.

18.Cheese Keto Cauliflower & Broccoli Rice

Ingredients

- 6 cups riced cauliflower
- 2 cup riced broccoli
- 2 tablespoon butter
- 1 teaspoon kosher salt
- 1/2 teaspoon ground black pepper
- 1/2 teaspoon garlic powder
- Pinch of ground nutmeg (x2)
- 1 cup shredded sharp cheddar cheese
- 1/2 cup mascarpone cheese

Preparation

- Combine all the ingredients, apart from the mascarpone cheese and cheddar cheese in bowl and microwave on high for about 4-5 minutes. Stir the mix.
- Add the cheddar cheese and microwave an additional 2 minutes. Add the mascarpone cheese until creamy and stir until fully incorporated.
- Mix well, check for seasoning, and enjoy!

19. Snowball bonbons a la Raffaello

Ingredients

- ¼ cup Almond flour
- ½ cup Coconut flour
- 6 oz (170 g) Cream cheese
- 2 oz (60g) Coconut oil
- Stevia or other no-calorie sweetener, the quantity depends on how sweet you like it, but be careful
- 1 cup Shredded unsweetened coconut
- 1 teaspoon Vanilla extract
- About 8-10 Macadamia nuts (this depends on how many snowballs you will make from the mixture)

Preparation

- Let the cream cheese and coconut oil to sit at room temperature to soften.
- Combine the almond flour, coconut flour, cream cheese, coconut oil and the sweetener in a bowl until a thick dough forms. If the mixture is too thick, or too runny, adjust with some more almond or coconut flour, or with cream cheese.
- Refrigerate for 10 minutes in the freezer.

- In the meantime, place shredded coconut and in a shallow plate.
- Remove the dough from freezer.
- Take a piece from the dough, place 1 macadamia nut and make the ball around it.
- Roll into the shredded coconut.
- Arrange on a baking sheet lined with parchment paper.
- Freeze the cookies for 10 to 30 minutes.
- Enjoy!

20.   Ovo-lacto

Ingredients

- 2 eggs
- 2 tablespoons shredded Parmesan cheese
- Oregano and basil, to taste, about 1 teaspoon
- Pinch of salt
- Pinch of black pepper
- 2 teaspoons olive oil
- 3 tablespoons sugar-free tomato sauce
- 2 ounces (56 g) Mozzarella cheese
- 1 tablespoon fresh basil

Preparation

- In a bowl, combine together the ingredients for the crust: the eggs, Parmesan cheese, basil, oregano, salt, black pepper. Whisk until well combined.
- Heat a skillet over medium high heat and drizzle with olive oil.
- Cook the crust for a several minutes until it's golden brown on both sides. The time will depend on your stove power, but maybe average 4-5 minutes per side. Watch out carefully

- Once the crust is done, line a baking dish with parchment paper and place the crust on it.
- Spread the sugar-free tomato toast on the crust. Add the mozzarella and bake in a preheated oven until the cheese melts down and becomes golden. Enjoy!

21. Keto pumpkin spice latte

Ingredients

- 1 shot espresso or brewed coffee
- ½ cup almond milk
- 2 tablespoons pumpkin puree
- 1 tablespoon full-fat coconut milk
- 2 tablespoons heavy whipping cream
- Cinnamon, to taste
- Pinch of nutmeg, to taste
- Cloves, to taste
- Cardamom, to taste
- Ginger, to taste
- Stevia or low-carb sweetener of choice
- 1 teaspoon vanilla extract

Optional for Even-More-Ketogenic-Latte:

- 1 teaspoon MCT Oil or Ghee Butter

Preparation

- Heat a sauce pan over low heat.
- Add the pumpkin puree and the spices – cinnamon, nutmeg, cloves, ginger, cardamom, and stir well.

- Stir constantly for 2 to 3 minutes, until mixture is fragrant.
- Add the milk and continue stirring. Cook until warm, but not boiling! When the mixture is warm, add in the stevia and the vanilla extract.
- Pour your coffee into a mug.
- Then pour the pumpkin-milk mixture over the coffee and top with heavy whipped cream.
- Sprinkle with cinnamon, if you wish.
- If you want, you can add the MCT oil or the butter to the coffee before adding the pumpkin-latte. Warm your soul with this delicious beverage!

22.   Healthy Avocado Fries

Ingredients

- 1 egg
- 1 avocado
- 1 ½ cup almond flour
- Crushed red pepper/chilli pepper
- Sea salt or Himalayan salt
- 1 tablespoon olive oil/coconut oil
- Mayonnaise,   for   serving

Preparation

- Preheat the oven to 450°F/230°C and line a baking dish with parchment paper.
- In a small bowl, scramble the egg.
- In another bowl, mix the almond flour, crushed red pepper or chilli peper (depending on how spicy you like it) and salt. Mix well.
- Slice the avocado into slices.
- Dip every avocado slice in the beaten egg first, and then immediately roll it into the almond flour mixture.
- Line the avocado "fries" on the parchment paper and drizzle with olive oil/coconut oil.

- Bake in the preheated oven for about 15 minutes or until golden.
- Serve with mayonnaise mixed with crushed red pepper, if desired. Enjoy!

23. Coconut Tuna Fish Cakes

Ingredients

- 2 cans of tuna fish in brine
- 2 eggs, scrambled
- Fresh basil, chopped
- 2 tablespoons of olive oil
- 2 tablespoons coconut shreds, unsweetened
- Chilli flakes, optional
- 2 tablespoons coconut flour
- Salt to taste
- 1 tablespoon coconut oil/coconut butter

Preparation

- Mix all the ingredients together in a bowl, except for the coconut oil/butter. Shape the mixture into patties.
- In a skillet on medium heat, add the coconut oil. Cook the patties until they turn golden. Turn them over and cook the other side until golden. Serve and enjoy!

24.   Keto coconut ice cream

Ingredients

- 2 cups coconut cream, full fat, no added sugar
- 1 cup heavy cream
- 6 egg yolks
- 3 tablespoons of (or by your taste and depending on how sweet you would like it to be) Stevia, Erythritol or low-calorie sweetener of choice
- 1 tablespoons of vanilla extract
- Cinnamon
- 3 tablespoons of shredded coconut
- Raspberries and blueberries for garnish (optional)
- Raw   cacao   nibs   for   garnish   (optional)

Instructions

- Beat the sweetener and egg yolks together with a mixer. Blend until homogeneous and creamy.
- In a medium pan, pour the beaten egg mixture over low medium heat. Add the vanilla extract, cinnamon, and heavy cream. Keep stirring until the ingredients are thoroughly mixed.
- When the edges of the mixture start to bubble, turn off the heat to avoid overcooking. Stir with the coconut cream

and some shredded coconut. Continually fold to create a thick, consistent custard texture.

- Freeze for 6-8 hours when the solution cools down to ambient temperature. Take it out from the freezer every two hours. To dissolve any ice crystals formed, mix with a spatula. Repeat at least twice for a smooth and crystal-free ice cream.

- When ready to serve, remove from the freezer. Top with some grated coconut, frozen raspberries, blueberries and crushed nibs of cacao, if you like. Love! Enjoy!

25.   Keto Asian beef salad

Ingredients

Sesame mayonnaise

- ¾ cup mayonnaise
- 1 tablespoon of sesame oil
- ½ tablespoon of lime juice
- salt and pepper

Beef

- 1 tablespoon of olive oil
- 1 tablespoon of fish sauce
- 1 tablespoon of grated fresh ginger
- 1 tablespoon of chili flakes
- 2/3 lb ribeye steaks

Salad

- 3 oz. Cherry tomatoes
- 2 oz. Cucumber
- 3 oz. Lettuce
- ½ red onion
- Fresh cilantro
- 1 tablespoon of sesame seeds
- 2 scallions

Preparation

- To prepare the sesame mayonnaise mix mayo with the sesame oil and lime juice. Season with salt and pepper. Put it aside.
- Mix all the beef marinade ingredients and pour them into a plastic bag. Add the beef and marinate at room temperature for 15 minutes or longer.
- Cut all salad vegetables, including scallions, into bite-sized pieces. Split between two plates.
- Heat a medium heat frying pan. Add the sesame seeds to the dry pan and toast for a few minutes or until browned and fragrant. Put it aside.
- Pat the meat with paper towels on both side. At high heat, sear on each side for a minute or two, then reduce heat to medium hot, cook until beef is medium, then move to a cutting board.
- Fry the scallions in the same pan for one minute.
- Slice the meat into thin slices across the grain. On top of the vegetables, put the beef and scallions.
- Serve with a dollop of sesame mayonnaise on the side and top with roasted sesame seeds.

26.   Keto Caprese omelet

Ingredients

- 6 eggs
- salt and pepper
- 1 tablespoon of chopped fresh basil or dried basil
- 2 tablespoons of olive oil
- 3 oz. cherry tomatoes cut in halves or tomatoes cut in slices
- 5 oz. fresh mozzarella cheese, diced or sliced

Preparation

- In a mixing bowl, crack the eggs, add salt and black pepper.
- Use a fork to whisk well until completely combined. Add basil and mix.
- In a large frying pan, heat the oil. Fry the tomatoes for a couple of minutes,.
- Fill the tomatoes with the egg batter. Before adding the mozzarella cheese, wait until the batter is slightly firm.
- Lower the heat and set the omelet. Serve and enjoy!

27.   Keto cheese roll-ups

Ingredients

- 8 oz. cheddar cheese or provolone cheese or edam cheese, in slices
- 2 oz. butter

Preparation

- On a large cutting board put the cheese slices.
- Slice butter with a cheese slicer or cut pieces that are really thin with a knife.
- Cover with butter every single cheese slice and roll it up. Serve like a treat.

28. Keto frittata with fresh spinach

Ingredients

- 5 oz. Diced bacon or chorizo
- 2 tablespoons of butter
- 8 oz. Fresh spinach
- 8 eggs
- 1 cup heavy whipping cream
- 5 oz. Shredded cheese
- Salt and pepper

Preparation

- Heat the oven to 175 ° C (350 ° F). Grease an individual ramekin or 9x9 baking dish.
- In medium heat, cook the bacon in butter until crispy. Add the spinach and stir until wilted. Remove the pan and set aside.
- Whisk together the eggs and milk and pour into the ramekins or baking dish.
- In the middle of the oven, add the bacon, spinach and cheese. Bake for 25–30 minutes or until set in the centre and golden brown on top.

29.   Keto pasta carbonara

Ingredients

- 1¼ cups heavy whipping cream
- 1 tablespoon of butter
- 10 oz. bacon or pancetta, diced
- ¼ cup mayonnaise
- salt and pepper
- 2 lbs zucchini
- 4 egg yolks
- 3 oz. grated parmesan cheese, some more for serving

Preparation

- Pour the heavy cream into a sauce pan over medium heat and bring to a boil. Reduce heat to medium low and let boil until it is reduced by a fourth for a few minutes.
- Melt the butter over medium heat in a large frying pan. Add bacon to the saucepan and fry until crispy. Put aside the bacon. Keep the fat warm at the bottom of the pan with low heat.
- Whisk the heavy cream with the mayonnaise. Salt and pepper to taste and cook until it warm. Reduce temperature to minimum, occasionally stirring.

- Make zucchini spirals with a spiralizer. If you don't have a spiralizer, you can use a potato peeler to make thin strips of zucchini.
- Put zoodles in a safe microwave bowl, and microwave it on high for 3-5 minutes, until hot, yet fresh and crispy. You can boil the zoodles in hot water for 30 seconds if you don't want to microwave.
- Mix the egg yolks, bacon and parmesan cheese in a separate bowl.
- Add bacon fat and hot cream sauce to the zoodles, stirring until the zoodles are fully covered. Make sure this mixture is slightly warm, then add the mixture of egg-bacon-parmesan cheese to the zoodles, tossing them all together (the egg mixture will scramble if it is too hot when combined).
- Split into four plates. Top with a generous amount of parmesan.

30.   Keto avocado, bacon and goat-cheese salad

Ingredients

- 8 oz. Goat cheese
- 8 oz. Bacon
- 2 avocados
- 4 oz. Arugula lettuce
- 4 oz. Walnuts
- Dressing
- 1 tablespoon of lemon, the juice
- ½ cup mayonnaise
- ½ cup olive oil
- 2 tablespoons of heavy whipping cream
- Salt and pepper

Preparation

- Preheat the oven to 200 ° C (400 ° F) and put parchment paper in a baking dish.
- Cut the goat's cheese into slices of about half inch (1 cm) and place it in the baking dish. Bake until the upper rack is golden.
- In a saucepan, fry the bacon until crispy.
- Cut the avocado into pieces and place the arugula on top. Add the goat cheese and the fried bacon. Sprinkle with nuts.

- Use an immersion blender to make the lemon juice, mayonnaise, olive oil and cream dressing. Season to taste with salt and pepper.

31. Keto smoked salmon plate

Ingredients

- ¾ Lb smoked salmon
- 1 cup mayonnaise
- 2 oz. Baby spinach
- 1 tablespoon of olive oil
- ½ lime (optional)
- Salt and pepper

Preparation

- On a plate, put the salmon, spinach, a wedge of lime, and a hearty dollop of mayonnaise.
- Sprinkle the spinach with olive oil and season with salt and pepper.

32.   Keto quesadillas

Ingredients

Low-carb tortillas

- 2 eggs
- 2 egg whites
- 6 oz. cream cheese
- ½ tablespoon of salt
- 1½ tablespoons of ground psyllium husk powder
- 1 tablespoon of coconut flour

Filling

- 1 tablespoon of olive oil or butter, for frying
- 5 oz. Mexican cheese or any hard cheese of your liking
- 1 oz. baby spinach

Filling

- 1 tablespoon of olive oil or butter, for frying
- 5 oz. Mexican cheese or any hard cheese of your liking
- 1 oz. baby spinach

Preparation

Tortillas

- Preheat the oven to a temperature of 200 ° C (400°F)

- Use an electric mixer to beat eggs and egg whites until fluffy. Add cream cheese and beat until the batter is smooth.
- Mix sugar, psyllium husk and coconut flour together in a pan. Mix well with each other.
- When beating, add the flour mixture to the batter. Let the batter rest for a couple of minutes when properly mixed. It should be as dense like pancake batter. Each step is influenced by your brand of psyllium husk powder — be patient... If it's not thickening enough, add more.
- Put parchment paper on a baking sheet. Use a spatula to spread the batter in a large rectangle over the parchment paper. You can cook them in a frying pan like pancakes if you want round tortillas.
- Bake for about 5–10 minutes or until the upper rack of the tortilla becomes crispy around the edges. Keep your eye on the oven — don't let the bottom of these delicious creations burn!
- Cut the big tortilla into smaller pieces (6 pieces per sheet of baking).

Quesadillas

- In a small, non-stick skillet, heat oil or butter over medium heat.

- Put tortilla and sprinkle with tomatoes, spinach and some more cheese in the frying pan. Top with a another tortilla.
- Fry each quesadilla on each side for about one minute. When the cheese melts, you'll know.

33.   Keto Asian cabbage stir-fry

Ingredients

- 1½ lbs green cabbage
- 4 oz. butter, divided
- 1 tablespoon of salt
- 1 tablespoon of onion powder
- ¼ tablespoon of ground black pepper
- 1 tablespoon of white wine vinegar
- 2 garlic cloves, minced
- 1 tablespoon of chili flakes
- 1 tablespoon of fresh ginger, finely chopped or grated
- 1¼ lbs ground beef
- 3 scallions, chopped in 1/2-inch slices
- 1 tablespoon of sesame oil
- Wasabi mayonnaise
- 1 cup mayonnaise
- ½ tablespoon of wasabi paste

Preparation

- Use a sharp knife or food processor to shred the cabbage.
- In a large frying pan, fry the cabbage in half of the butter or wok pan over moderate to high heat. Softening the cabbage can take a while, but don't let it turn brown.

- Apply vinegar and spices. Stir and fry for a few more minutes. Place the chicken in a pan.
- In the same frying pan, melt the remaining butter. Remove garlic, ginger and chili flakes. Sauté for a couple of minutes.
- Add ground meat and brown until the meat is cooked thoroughly and most juices have evaporated. Reduce the heat a little bit.
- Add scallions and cabbage to the meat.Stir until it's all hot. Add salt and pepper to taste. Before serving, sprinkle with sesame oil.
- Mix with the wasabi mayonnaise with a small amount of wasabi and add more until the taste is perfect. Serve the hot stir-fry with a wasabi mayonnaise dollop on top.

34. Keto pancakes with berries and whipped cream

Ingredients

Pancakes

- 4 eggs
- 7 oz. cottage cheese
- 1 tablespoon of ground psyllium husk powder
- 2 oz. butter or coconut oil

Toppings

- 2 oz. fresh raspberries or fresh blueberries or fresh strawberries
- 1 cup heavy whipping cream

Preparation

- In a medium-sized pan, add eggs, cottage cheese and psyllium husk and blend. Let it thicken a little for 5-10 minutes.
- In a non-stick pan, melt butter or oil. Fry the pancakes on medium-low heat on each side for 3–4 minutes. Don't make them too wide or they're going to be difficult to flip.
- In a separate bowl, add cream and whip until soft peaks are formed.

- Serve the pancakes with your choice of whipped cream and berries

35. Pork chops with green beans and garlic butter

Ingredients

- Garlic butter
- 5 oz. Butter, at room temperature
- ½ tablespoon of garlic powder
- 1 tablespoon of dried parsley
- 1 tablespoon of lemon juice
- Salt and pepper
- Pork chops
- 4 pork chops
- 2 oz. Butter, for frying
- 1 lb fresh green beans
- Salt and pepper

Preparation

- Mix the butter, garlic, lemon juice and parsley. Season to taste, use salt and pepper. Deposit back.
- Make a few tiny cuts in the fat around the chops to help them stay flat before frying. Mix with pepper and salt.
- Melt the butter in a large frying pan over medium to high heat. Remove the chops and fry on each side for about 5 minutes, or until golden brown and cooked thoroughly.
- Take the chops off the pan and keep warm.

- Use the same pan to pour in the beans. Season with salt and pepper. Cook over medium - high heat until the beans have a vibrant colour, and are slightly softened but still a little crunchy.
- Serve the pork chops and beans with a dollop of melting garlic butter on top.

36. Keto hamburger patties with creamy tomato sauce and fried cabbage

Ingredients

Hamburger patties

- 1½ lbs ground beef
- 1 egg
- 3 oz. crumbled feta cheese
- 1 tablespoon of salt
- ¼ tablespoon of ground black pepper
- 2 oz. fresh parsley, finely chopped
- 1 tablespoon of olive oil, for frying
- 2 tablespoons of butter, for frying

Gravy

- ¾ Cup heavy whipping cream
- 1 oz. Fresh parsley, coarsely chopped
- 2 tablespoon of tomato paste or ajvar relish
- Salt and pepper
- Fried green cabbage
- 1½ lbs shredded green cabbage
- 4½ oz. Butter
- Salt and pepper

Preparation

Hamburger patties and gravy

- Pour all the hamburger ingredients into a large bowl. Mix it with a wooden spoon, or clean hands. Don't over-mix as that can make your patties hard. Using wet hands to form 8 oblong patties.
- Fill a large frying pan with butter and olive oil. Fry for at least 10 minutes over medium - high heat, or until the patties have turned a nice colour. Flip them in for even cooking a few times.
- Whisk the tomato paste and the milk together in a small bowl. When the patties are almost done, add this mixture to the saucepan. Remove for a few minutes and allow to simmer. Season with salt and pepper.
- Sprinkle on top of chopped parsley before serving.

Butter-fried green cabbage

- Finely cut the cob with a food processor or a sharp knife.
- Add a large frying pan with oil.
- Position the saucepan over medium heat and sauté the shredded cob for at least 15 minutes or until the cob is wilted and golden brown around the edges.
- Regularly swirl and slightly lower heat towards the top. Season with salt and pepper.

37.   Keto coconut porridge

Ingredients

- 1 egg, beaten
- 1 tablespoon of coconut flour
- 1 pinch ground psyllium husk powder
- 1 pinch salt
- 1 oz. butter or coconut oil
- 4 tablespoons of coconut cream

Preparation

- Mix the seeds, coconut flour, psyllium husk powder and salt in a small bowl.
- Melt the butter and the coconut cream over low heat. Slowly whisk in the combination of ingredients, mixing until smooth, dense texture is obtained.
- Serve with a cream or coconut milk. Place a few fresh or frozen berries over your porridge and enjoy

38.   Keto shrimp and artichoke plate

Ingredients

- 4 eggs
- 10 oz. Cooked and peeled shrimp
- 14 oz. Canned artichokes
- 6 sun-dried tomatoes in oil
- ½ cup mayonnaise
- 1½ oz. Baby spinach
- 4 tablespoons of olive oil
- Salt and pepper

Preparation

- Have the eggs fried. Carefully lower them into boiling water and boil for 4-8 minutes, depending on whether you like soft or hard boiled.
- Freeze the eggs in ice-cold water for 1-2 minutes after they are done; this will make extracting the shell easier.
- Put on a plate bacon, shrimps, artichokes, mayonnaise, sun-dried tomatoes and spinach;
- Drizzle the spinach with olive oil Season to taste, and finish with salt and pepper.

39. Keto ribeye steak with oven-roasted vegetables

Ingredients

- 1 lb broccoli
- 1 whole garlic
- 10 oz. Cherry tomatoes
- 3 tablespoons of olive oil
- 1 tablespoon of dried thyme or dried oregano or dried basil
- 1½ lbs ribeye steaks
- Salt and pepper
- Anchovy butter
- 1 oz. Anchovies
- 5 oz. Butter, at room temperature
- 1 tablespoon of lemon juice
- Salt and pepper

Preparation

- Make the butter with anchovies. The anchovy fillets are finely chopped and combined with butter (at room temperature), lemon juice, salt and pepper. Deposit aside.
- Preheat the oven to 225 ° C (450 ° F) and make sure your meat is out of the refrigerator before cooking to reach

room temperature. Divide the garlic into cloves but don't cut them. Slice the broccoli into florets. You can also include them in stem, just peel and slice off any rough parts.

- Grease a broad roasting saucepan and put the vegetables in one plate. Spray on finish and drizzle with olive oil. Place the roasting pan in the oven for 15 minutes and give it a touch to paint.

- Brush the olive oil into the meat and season with salt and pepper. Quickly cook in a frying pan on high heat. You're just looking at giving the meat a good sewn surface at this stage.

- Remove the pan from the oven and make room among the vegetables for the beef.

- Reduce the heat to 200 ° C (400 ° F) and put the pan back in the oven for up to 10 to 15 minutes, depending on how you like your meat-rare, medium or well-done.

- Remove from the oven, and place on each piece of meat a dollop of anchovy butter. Directly serve.

40. Keto prosciutto-wrapped asparagus with goat cheese

Ingredients

- 12 pieces of green asparagus
- 2 oz. prosciutto, in thin slices
- 5 oz. goat cheese
- ¼ tablespoon of ground black pepper
- 2 tablespoons of olive oil

Preparation

- Preheat your oven to 450 ° F (225 ° C) with broiler feature ideally on.
- Drain asparagus, then cut it.
- Slice the cheese into 12 pieces, then split each slice into 2 pieces.
- Cut the prosciutto slices lengthwise into two pieces, and wrap each piece around one asparagus and two pieces of cheese.
- Put in a parchment lined baking dish. Add pepper and olive oil to drizzle.
- Broil in the oven, until golden brown for about 15 minutes.

442

CONCLUSION

Credit for having mastered the ketogenic diet. Now, you can lose excess body weights, live healthily, and have sufficient body energy for your daily work. Although doing all of these will not be an easy task, it's important to consider how best to keep up with your new health status.

Maintaining weight loss can be easier than losing body weight. Sure, one might be tempted when trying to reduce body weight to take up the meals that were missed off. Often, when one stops taking the keto diet, the metabolism changes (slows down) and keeping weight loss is difficult.

Almost definitely you wouldn't want to return to an unhealthy lifestyle that depends on high sugar, carbohydrates and grains. The above tips can therefore motivate you to maintain a healthy life for your new ones.

Consider the options before leaving the ketogenic diet. Have a strategy on the table, and move towards its completion. With the various options offered on a keto diet, changes to a replacement eating method will be smooth.

CPSIA information can be obtained
at www.ICGtesting.com
Printed in the USA
LVHW050728241120
672556LV00003B/32